Therapy Ball
Workbook

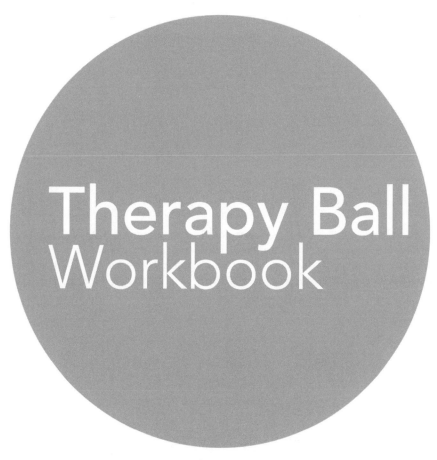

Therapy Ball
Workbook

Illustrated Step-by-Step Guide to Stretching,
Strengthening and Rehabilitative Techniques

Dr. Karl Knopf

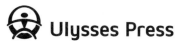

Ulysses Press

Published in the United States by
Ulysses Press
P.O. Box 3440
Berkeley, CA 94703
www.ulyssespress.com

ISBN: 978-1-61243-299-1
Library of Congress Control Number 2013922722

Printed in the United States by United Graphics

10 9 8 7 6 5 4 3 2 1

Acquisitions: Kelly Reed
Managing editor: Claire Chun
Editor: Lily Chou
Proofreader: Elyce Berrigan-Dunlop
Indexer: Sayre Van Young
Production: Jake Flaherty
Cover design: what!design @ whatweb.com
Photographs: © Rapt Productions except on page 6 © marema/shutterstock.com
Models: Michael Ciociola, Nadia Velasquez
Make-up: Sabrina Foster

Distributed by Publishers Group West

Please Note
This book has been written and published strictly for informational purposes, and in no way should be used as a substitute for actual instruction with qualified professionals. The author and publisher are providing you with information in this work so that you can have the knowledge and can choose, at your own risk, to act on that knowledge. The author and publisher also urge all readers to be aware of their health status and to consult health care professionals before beginning any health program.

contents

PART 1

overview

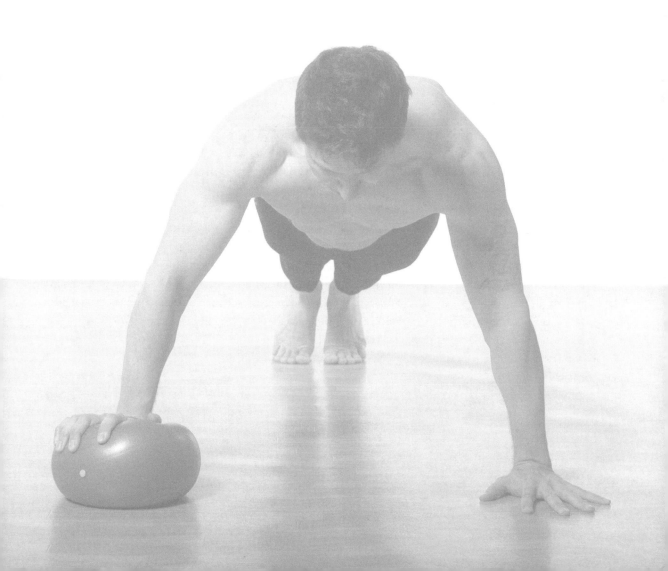

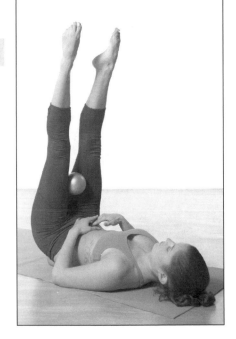

introduction

Pain is the great equalizer, whether we're rich or poor, fit or unfit, young or old. Acute pain can cripple you while chronic pain can devastate you. Pain is the main complaint for 40 percent of visits to the family physician. Only 50 percent of those visits have satisfactory outcomes, leaving patients wondering what the cause id and what they can do.

Sometimes poor posture and improper body mechanics, along with overtraining specific muscles, lead to increased muscle tension and harmful body alignment. Other times trauma to an area can intensify muscle tension, which can contribute to muscle spasms. If these dysfunctions aren't addressed properly, they can lead to reduced mobility and chronic physical problems. Frequently there's no "cure" for the pain, only ways to manage it. The key is to find a method that provides the most benefit for the least amount of risk.

The therapy ball is considered one of those options.

Each of us has our own unique threshold for pain. Although there's no universal cure-all that can rid us of these physical annoyances for good, there are many options, such as medication and massage, that can ease our discomfort. There are even methods we can apply ourselves. You've probably used a foam roller to loosen tight hamstrings, release your back, and improve your balance. Did you know that the balls you play with, anything from golf balls to basketballs, can provide

the same benefits, in addition to keeping your heart healthy?

With therapy balls, you can roll your way to better health! *Therapy Ball Workbook* explains how you can use practically any ball—large or small, soft or hard—as a "therapy ball." It also presents exercises for physical rehab, core strengthening, posture correction, general conditioning, self-massage and stress relief—all ways to maintain a flexible, strong body and prevent future injury.

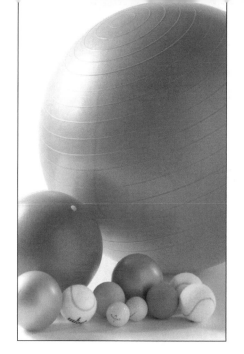

what's a therapy ball?

There are a few balls on the market earmarked for massage therapy and a number that actually call themselves "fitness" and "therapy" balls. However, as far as *Therapy Ball Workbook* is concerned, no single type of ball is the "perfect" therapy ball. In fact, most balls used for general fitness and recreation can be repurposed for therapy, be it massage, rehab or conditioning. The size, shape and density of the ball you select should be determined by the goal of your session and, if applicable, the area of your body you aim to address.

In general, small balls (between 1 to 6 inches) with some give, such as tennis balls and softballs, are good candidates for self-massage and muscle release. If your muscles require a firmer touch, try denser balls such as those used in golf and lacrosse. Smaller balls have the benefit of getting into areas that other tools (pressure point wand, foam rollers) have a hard time reaching.

Balls with some give can also be used for core strengthening and conditioning—the squishier the ball, the more unstable it usually is. The stability ball (also known as the Swiss or Pilates ball) is a popular core-strengthening tool and perhaps the best known of the therapy balls. It comes in several sizes and can be inflated to your desired firmness. You might also see mini versions of the stability ball (often called "fitness," "therapy" and "yoga" balls) used in Pilates and core-training classes. These balls typically run 4 to 10 inches and are often kept underinflated.

Some specialized balls have knobs and nubs to stimulate circulation, which work well for the hands and feet. Others have bumpy surfaces to promote sensory stimulation, while those with a hard, smooth surface are designed to be held in your hands to provide better trigger-point tension relief. These specialty balls may be found at sporting-goods, yoga, Pilates and physical therapy stores.

The nice thing about using balls for therapy is that you probably have at least one lying around the house. If not, they're reasonably priced or even free (say, around your local tennis court or golf course) and a good, all-purpose health tool.

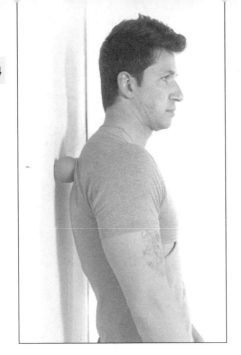

why use therapy balls?

Too often in the world of fitness, people focus on developing stronger muscles or improving performance in a sport but neglect the subtler aspects of fitness such as stretching and flexibility. Most exercise programs and sports place emphasis on one particular muscle group, thus causing muscle imbalances that create more inflexibility.

The key to staying healthy and functional is to understand the interplay between all the characteristics of the body that are critical to optimal fitness, function and wellness. Being too strong and tight is just as bad as being too flexible. Our bodies are like a symphony; each part has a special role that needs to be played at the correct time and be well tuned in order to produce a beautiful harmony.

It's very difficult for the average fitness buff to understand the delicate relationship between dose and response. Too many people believe that more and harder is always better. It's the enlightened person who understands the balance between physical activity, rest and mindful movements. The longer I work with people of all levels, the more I realize that having a firm yet supple body is the key to achieving functional fitness and a pain-free life. Whether you're sedentary or very active, a daily routine of stretching and muscle relaxation is critical in preventing joint dysfunctions and chronic pain.

Therapy balls are wonderful, versatile tools that can improve mobility and flexibility, prevent possible injury and release muscular tension while also adding diversity to your standard exercise program.

Tennis, golf, lacrosse and softballs are perhaps most commonly used for self-massage, the goal of which is to break up interwoven muscle fibers and help move oxygenated blood into the muscles. Softer, squishier balls, when used during common exercises like push-ups and back extensions, provide an unstable surface that challenges the central nervous system to maintain control. Simply squeezing a squishy ball between your knees during an abdominal curl-up engages more core muscles and reinforces the interconnectedness between the muscles.

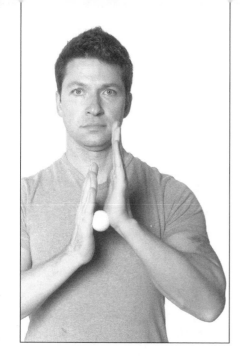

therapy balls and self-massage

The therapy ball is a wonderful self-help tool to reduce muscle tightness and provide deep muscle massage and pressure release. The advantage that the therapy ball has over other self-massage tools is that it can provide a multi-directional massage to the area in need (similar to what a massage therapist would do), or simply be held in place until a trouble spot releases (like what you'd encounter with an acupressurist).

Oftentimes a simple injury such as a muscle strain or contusion can contribute to muscle knots or "trigger points"—small patches of super-contracted muscle fibers that cause aching and stiffness. These trigger points can affect the performance of the whole muscle and spread pain to adjacent areas (called "referred pain"). In addition, a person who has an injury typically "guards" the area/joint, which often leads to reduced range of motion in that area and further dysfunction.

There are approximately 620 potential trigger points in our muscles. These trigger points reportedly show up in the same places in every person (the chart on page 6 highlights the most common trigger points). In an active trigger point, pain or tenderness can either be felt locally or in another location ("referred pain"). If you pay attention to your body, you'll notice that certain locations feel painful when pressed while others don't. A latent trigger point is one that exists but doesn't yet refer pain. However, a

latent trigger point can influence muscle activation patterns, which can result in poor muscle coordination and balance.

Many people call active trigger points "ouch" points, whereby just pushing on the point elicits pain. When trigger points are present in muscles, there's often pain and weakness in areas a distance from where the pain is. It's suggested that applying pressure to trigger points can release tension, reduce stress and promote wellness. While these methods are not a substitute

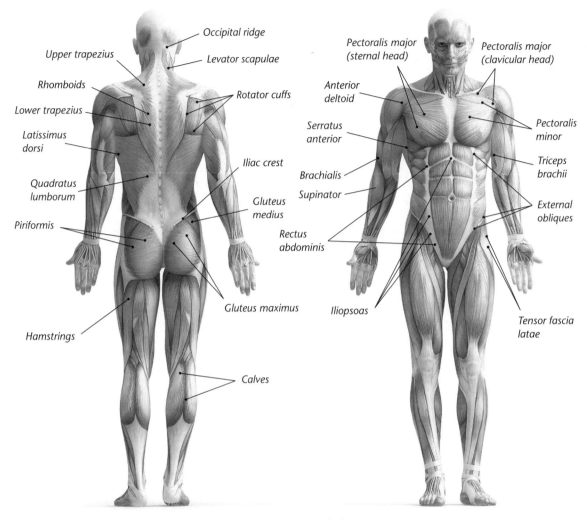

Upper trapezius

Rhomboids

Lower trapezius

Latissimus dorsi

Quadratus lumborum

Piriformis

Hamstrings

Occipital ridge

Levator scapulae

Rotator cuffs

Iliac crest

Gluteus medius

Gluteus maximus

Calves

Pectoralis major (sternal head)

Pectoralis major (clavicular head)

Anterior deltoid

Serratus anterior

Brachialis

Supinator

Rectus abdominis

Iliopsoas

Pectoralis minor

Triceps brachii

External obliques

Tensor fascia latae

Common Trigger Points

for Western medicine, they often can be used in a complementary manner.

Other factors are believed to lead to muscle stiffness and soreness. One theory is that when soft tissue gets injured, the fascia (thin connective tissue that surrounds muscles) does not slide freely. Performing myofascial techniques along with a systematic stretching routine can facilitate the break-up of these adhesions.

While this book is not intended as a replacement for physical therapy or a trained massage therapist, it can be a great complement to a home-based post-rehab routine or preventive program, used in concert with your therapist's input.

However, since so many things contribute to tightness and soreness, it's always wise to consult with your health professional before performing a self-massage. Keep in mind that pain is your body's panel light letting you know something isn't perfect, thus always make sure there's no significant health issue causing your pain.

How to Use Therapy Balls for Self-Massage

Learning to tune in to the parts of your body that are tight is the first step in correcting any physical dysfunction stemming from muscle imbalance. Which activities do you participate in that contribute to your tightness? Is it too much of one kind of exercise or too much time spent hunched over a desk? A regular therapy ball program that addresses those tight areas, coupled with proper body mechanics, would be a wise investment.

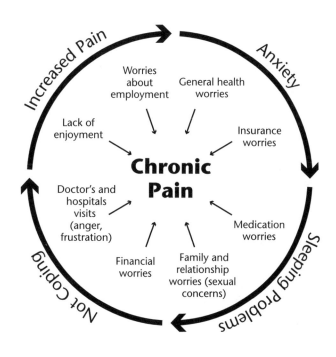

Chronic Pain

Increased Pain / Anxiety / Sleeping Problems / Not Coping

Worries about employment — General health worries — Insurance worries — Medication worries — Family and relationship worries (sexual concerns) — Financial worries — Doctor's and hospitals visits (anger, frustration) — Lack of enjoyment

Most balls are placed under specific locations and either held in place for a certain amount of time or rolled over back and forth, depending on your tolerance. While holding the ball over the pressure point might not feel great, the relief that follows after you've broken apart those adhesions will pleasantly surprise you. Most trigger point experts suggest the following:

- Relax the targeted muscles prior to a session either by using a hold-relax muscle stretch or a warm shower.
- Avoid circulatory locations such as behind the knee, armpit and neck.
- Only take the pressure intensity to a 5 or 6 on your pain scale of 10.
- Apply pressure to the area for only 8 to 20 seconds, or as tolerated.

- You're unique—follow your instincts.

The key to achieving a desirable outcome is to know when to press hard, when to press gently and when to avoid an area completely. Keep in mind that each body part requires different amounts of pressure. Start with a light touch and move to deeper pressure. The lower legs are often very sensitive, whereas the back, buttocks and shoulders often can tolerate a different level of pressure. Use caution when doing anything around the abdominal area, or if you have any health issues. It's wise to consult your physician before engaging in abdominal therapy ball moves.

Many times the more fit or tense you are, the more uncomfort-able the "hold" can be, so consider starting with a softer ball, a shorter duration or a lighter intensity. The bottom line is that ball selection is a personal choice. If you feel better after the session, the type of ball used was correct. Listen to your body! Each of us has a different threshold for discomfort. Aim for an experience that "hurts so good." Be intuitive about the positioning and the amount of pressure you exert.

If you allow too much time to lapse between sessions, the adhesions reform and then you have to start over. A little bit of self-massage done regularly is far more beneficial than a lot done seldomly.

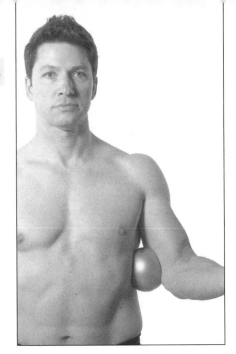

self-assessment of flexibility

Through testing, you can hone in on your problem areas and maximize your ability to design an effective therapy ball routine. One easy way is to ask someone you feel comfortable with to gently press various trigger points on your body while you register the level of discomfort you notice. You might hardly notice the pressure in some areas while others elicit an unexpected "ouch!"

Many of our chronic muscle imbalances are a result of tight hamstrings and upper back muscles as well as hip flexors. Checking out your posture is a simple way to see if how you stand and move is a possible cause of your discomfort. The following simple fitness tests will check for muscle tightness and poor flexibility in the most problematic areas of the body for most people—the lower back, hamstrings and shoulders. (Tight hamstrings, incidentally, are a common contributor to lower back pain.) These assessments are gross evaluations and should be a launching point for discussion with your health professional; they're not intended for diagnosis.

Posture Test

Stand in front of a mirror and, if possible, have a series of horizontal and vertical lines behind you. This may sound silly, but placing dots on your shoulders, hips and knees can help highlight any postural shifts.

While facing the mirror, check for the following:

- Is one shoulder higher than the other?
- Is one hip higher than the other?
- Is your chin directly over your sternum?
- Is your sternum over your belly button?
- Is your weight evenly distributed over both feet?

Your shoulders and hips should be level, your chin should be centered over your sternum, your sternum should be aligned over your belly button and your weight should be evenly distributed over both feet. If they're not, consider your body mechanics: Do you always carry your bag/briefcase over the same shoulder? Do you favor one leg over another? You may need to change your movement patterns or consult a physical therapist to bring proper alignment back to your body.

Now take a look at yourself from the side and check for the following (be sure to assess both sides):

- Are your ears over the middle of your shoulders?
- Is there a significant arch in your lower back or is it flat?
- Are your hips over your knees and ankles?

Your ears should be aligned with your shoulders, your lower back should have a slight arch and your hips should be over your knees and ankles. Again, if your alignment is off, you may need to change your movement patterns or consult a physical therapist to bring proper alignment back to your body.

Alternate Posture Test

Stand with your back to the wall with your heels 3 to 5 inches from the wall and your rear end against the wall. Now ask yourself:

- Are my shoulder blades flat against the wall?
- Is there a significant arch in my lower back?
- Is the back of my head comfortably touching the wall?

- Can I place my hands on my shoulders and touch my elbows to the wall?

Ideally you should be able to place your hands on your shoulder and touch your elbows to the wall. Most men can't because their shoulder and chest region is too tight. Thus meaning they need to stretch the chest area. If your hips are pushed significantly forward or back, creating a significantly arched or flat back, they can contribute to lower back discomfort.

If you notice significant misalignment, consider focusing on improving flexibility in the areas that are tight. Proceed with the following tests to help determine where those areas are.

Hamstring Test

Sit on the floor with your legs straight out in front of you and your toes pointing up. While keeping your back straight, place your hands on top of each other and extend your arms forward, reaching for your toes.

- If you can touch your toes, fair.
- If you can reach past your toes, great.
- If you can't reach your toes, you need to work on improving flexibility and mobility in your lower back and the backs of your thighs.

Shoulder Flexibility Test

Stand tall, reach your right hand to the ceiling and then bend your arm to let your arm fall behind your head. Reach your left hand up your back and attempt to touch the fingers of your right hand—don't force it! Do both sides.

- If your fingers touch, fair.
- If your fingers overlap, great.
- If your fingers don't touch, you need to work on shoulder and chest flexibility.

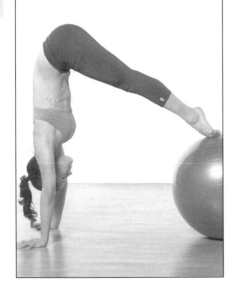

before you begin

To the world you are one person but to one person you may be the world. Treat yourself kindly! Therapy balls are a wonderful way to improve mobility and release muscular tension while adding diversity and challenge to your exercise program. Still, it's always advised to seek professional input if you're pregnant, have a pre-existing condition, are in poor health or severe pain, have osteoporosis and/or have poor range of motion/flexibility (see the flexibility assessments on page 8).

The key to effective use of therapy balls lies in the following concepts:

- Understand how long and how much pressure is correct for you.
- Be relaxed and warm. Dress in clothes that allow you freedom of movement.
- Understand the interconnectedness of your muscles (e.g., tight hamstrings influence lower back pain).
- Learn which order of positions is best for you (e.g., large muscle groups followed by isolated muscles).
- Don't go beyond mild discomfort—pain causes tightness.

You should feel better when you release. Never hold a position too long or hard!

- Be patient; don't expect overnight results. You don't need to hold a position to the point of pain.
- Avoid any area that has been injured until cleared by your doctor.
- Never perform therapy ball moves over an area where inflammation or swelling is present.
- Don't perform therapy ball moves directly over a bony area or areas where you can feel your pulse, like the sides of your

neck, under your armpit and behind your knee.

- If you experience soreness that lasts more than 24 hours, re-evaluate the routine.
- Never self-diagnose yourself— pain is your body's warning system. Always seek medical advice. Sometimes referred pain in your back could be a heart attack.
- Never do too much too soon.
- When lying on a therapy ball, align your spine correctly and never compromise your balance.

PART 2

programs

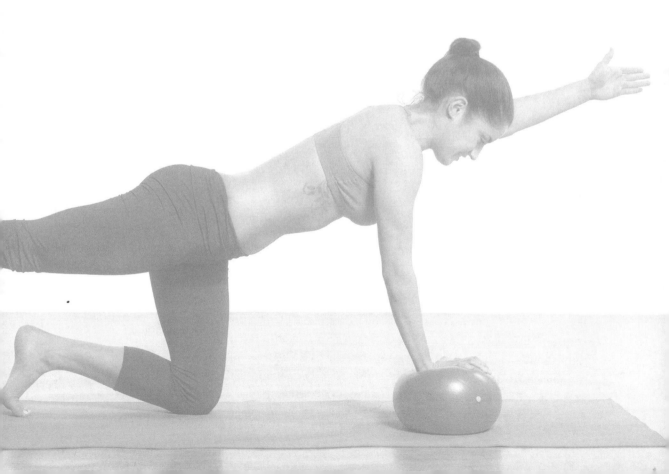

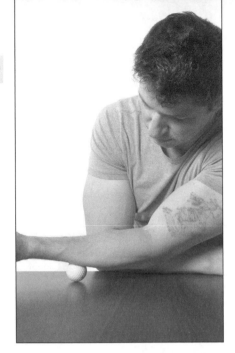

how to use this book

This section features several programs that address a variety of needs, from self-massage to core strengthening to stretching. Detailed instructions on how to perform the movements can be found in Part 3. Feel free to choose one of these programs and perform it as noted, or add any exercises from Part 3 as you see fit.

Keep in mind that using a therapy ball may look like child's play but utilizing it correctly to obtain an ideal response is no easy feat. If you've been diagnosed with a medical condition, it's highly recommended that you obtain personalized instruction from a trained therapist prior to engaging in any of these programs or exercises. This book should be used in concert with your health provider to assist you to a better-balanced body. Your body, just like a spinning top, functions best when all the forces are in sync.

Frequently Asked Questions

If you prefer to create your own routine, these FAQs will help you put together the workout that best fits your needs.

How Much Space Do I Need?

You only need the amount of space it takes for you to stand/sit/lie down with your therapy ball and spread your arms. The beauty of using therapy balls is that they're easy to carry and can be used anywhere: the floor in front of your TV, out on the lawn, at the gym, even sitting at your desk.

Which Ball Should I Use?

Selecting the right ball for your needs and goals is a personal decision, but there are certain tips you should keep in mind. In general, firmer balls such as tennis and softballs are best for pressure release and self-massage. Harder balls, like those used in golf and lacrosse, can also be used but they'll be much more intense. For core strengthening and conditioning, you'll typically use a ball with some give (we'll call these "stability" balls), like the popular large ball or smaller fitness ball. Depending on the exercise, an underinflated ball may provide more challenge than a firmly inflated one—you'll have to (safely) experiment to find the right one for you. Regardless of the firmness of the ball, make sure that the ball is safe for your body weight and avoid sharp objects.

When Should I Do the Exercises/ Self-Massage?

Aim to perform your therapy ball session several times a week but avoid doing it shortly after a meal.

Make therapy ball time a special time for you to relax, refresh and renew yourself!

How Do I Select Which Exercises to Do?

An ancient physician once told his medical students, "If you listen to your patients they will tell you their cure, so it is with you." That said, if you truly listen to your body, it will tell you which exercises are correct for you. For instance, a difficult day sitting over a computer will necessitate a different set of self-massage movements than a day of yard work.

In general, try to do at least one movement/exercise that addresses all the major muscle groups daily. Spend a little extra time on trouble spots as needed.

When doing self-massage, try to start at the proximal (top) parts of the body or limb. For example, start at the top of your leg and move toward your foot. Use larger, softer balls before progressing to smaller, firmer balls.

Do not perform self-massage if you have or are experiencing any of the following:

- Acute sprain/strain or skin lesions
- Skin diseases
- An unhealed fracture or wound
- Osteoporosis, fibromyaglia
- Edema, a bleeding disorder, or a vascular or heart condition

If you feel worse after a session, consider reducing the intensity and the duration of your next session. The 2-hour rule is a great suggestion: If you feel better 2 hours post-session, then what you did is probably right for you. However, if you wake up in the morning with more aches and pains, re-evaluate the moves.

How Many Reps of the Exercises Should I Do?

Start with only one set at a light intensity and duration and see how your body responds. Don't focus on duration or number of times; trust your body to be your guide. Be kind to yourself. Two to five times is

generally a safe starting point for conditioning exercises. There are infinite possibilities—just listen to your body.

How Long Should I Apply Pressure during Self-Massage Sessions?

When performing self-massage, keep the movements small and gentle and progress as appropriate. Don't apply too much pressure at first. Focus on areas of tension; no particular direction or amount of pressure is right or wrong. Breathe deeply and exhale the tension: Inhale slowly either through your nose or mouth fully for a count of 4 to 6 and then exhale slowly through your lips (as if blowing out a candle) for a count of 8 to 12. You may enjoy a glass of water after each session to cleanse out toxins released by your muscles.

To achieve ideal results, try to give yourself 10 to 30 minutes daily to quiet your mind and relax your body. Think about the areas of your body that feel like they need attention and select moves/positions accordingly. It might be best to only do 2 or 3 positions and hold them a little longer than try to cram many moves into a routine. I also like to blend trigger-point holds with a stretch. Performing self-massage several times a day might be better than one long session. If you feel worse 2 hours post-session or the next day, adjust the variables of your next session.

THERAPY BALL SUGGESTIONS

In Part 3, we recommend the types of balls to be used in the various exercises. Here are the categories and the most common balls of their type.

Small firm *(less than 4" in diameter)*: tennis, racquetball

Medium firm *(4" to 10" in diameter)*: rubber playground (think "four square")

Small hard *(less than 4" in diameter)*: golf, lacrosse

Medium hard *(4" to 10" in diameter)*: medicine, basketball

Small stability *(less than 4" in diameter)*: soft fitness

Medium stability *(4" to 10" in diameter)*: soft fitness

Large stability: standard Pilates, Swiss

This routine is designed to acquaint you with the ball. While performing this program, evaluate how you're able to move about and still maintain your balance. This is a fine program to address overall core stability. If possible, perform this series 2 to 3 times a week. Remember, the quality of the motion is more important than the time or reps. Once you accomplish the suggested reps/duration, do 2 to 3 sets.

START-UP ROUTINE

EXERCISE	BALL	DURATION
Ball Sit Orientation *page 51*	large stability	2–120 sec
Seated Hip Movement *page 52*	large stability	2–30 sec
Ball Sit with Foot Lift *page 54*	large stability	3–10 reps
Ball Sit with Leg Extension *page 55*	large stability	3–15 reps
Ball Sit with Leg Extension & Arm Raise *page 56*	large stability	3–15 reps
Pelvic Lift *page 25*	small firm or stability	5–60 sec
Pelvic Lift with Arm Lift *page 58*	medium firm, hard or stability	5–20 reps
Pelvic Lift with Leg Extension *page 59*	medium firm, hard or stability	5–20 reps
Pelvic Lift with Arm Lift & Leg Extension *page 60*	medium firm, hard or stability	5–20 reps

core stability workout

This program is designed to challenge your core quickly and can be performed before or after a workout, or even as a stand-alone routine. If you perform this routine, consider doing the Back Strengthening Workout (page 16) the day after. Remember, the quality of the motion is more important than the time or reps. Once you accomplish the suggested reps/duration, do 2 to 3 sets.

CORE STABILITY WORKOUT		
EXERCISE	**BALL**	**DURATION**
Leg Extension *page 22*	small firm or stability	5–15 reps
Pelvic Lift *page 25*	small firm or stability	5–15 reps
Arm/Leg Combination *page 27*	small firm or stability	5–15 reps
Curl-Up *page 28*	small firm or stability	3–10 reps
Back-on-Ball Crunch *page 30*	large stability	2–10 reps

back strengthening workout

This program is designed to address the posterior muscles of the core quickly and can be performed before or after a workout, or even as a stand-alone routine. If you perform this routine, consider doing the Core Stability Workout (page 15) the day after. Remember, the quality of the motion is more important than the time or reps. Once you accomplish the suggested reps/duration, do 2 to 3 sets.

BACK STRENGTHENING WORKOUT

EXERCISE	BALL	DURATION
I, Y & T *page 37*	large stability	3–5 reps
Double-Arm Lift *page 39*	large stability	3–5 reps
Double-Leg Lift *page 40*	large stability	3–5 reps
Prone Arm & Leg Lift *page 41*	large stability	3–5 reps
Superman *page 42*	large stability	2–5 reps
Stability Ball Plank *page 43*	medium or large stability	5–30 sec
Back Extension *page 38*	large stability	3–5 reps

total torso tune-up

This program focuses on developing a strong and solid abdominal region. If you're very lean, you may even notice a six pack after a while. Remember, the quality of the motion is more important than the time or reps. Once you accomplish the suggested reps/duration, do 2 to 3 sets.

TOTAL TORSO TUNE-UP		
EXERCISE	**BALL**	**DURATION**
Arm Swing *page 26*	small firm or stability	3–10 reps
Curl-Up *page 28*	small firm or stability	3–15 reps
Back-on-Ball Crunch *page 30*	large stability	3–15 reps
Back-on-Ball Twisting Crunch *page 31*	large stability	3–15 reps
Back-on-Ball Leg Lift *page 35*	large stability	3–15 reps
Alternating Curl-Up *page 36*	small or firm stability	3–10 reps
Supine Stability Orientation *page 29*	large stability	10–120 sec
Supine Marching *page 32*	large stability	10–120 sec
Supine Stability—Arms *page 33*	large stability	3–15 reps
Supine Stability—Legs *page 34*	large stability with small firm or stability	3–15 reps
Double-Leg Lift *page 40*	large stability	1–5 reps
Leg Circle *page 23*	small stability	1–5 reps
Heel Slide *page 24*	small firm or stability	1–5 reps

total-body workout

This routine will give you a total-body workout, with upper-body conditioning and core-stability exercises as well as lower-extremity toning. Remember, the quality of the motion is more important than the time or reps. Once you accomplish the suggested reps/duration, do 2 to 3 sets.

TOTAL-BODY WORKOUT		
EXERCISE	**BALL**	**DURATION**
Push-Up *page 44*	medium or large stability	1–20 reps
Ball Switch Push-Up *page 45*	medium stability or firm	1–20 reps
Plank to Pike *page 46*	large stability	1–15 reps
Plank to Side Salutation *page 47*	large stability	1–10 reps
Reverse Trunk Curl *page 48*	large stability	1–10 reps
Arm Pointer *page 49*	medium firm, hard or stability	3–15 reps
Bird Dog *page 50*	medium firm, hard or stability	10–120 sec
Inner Thigh Toner *page 61*	small firm or stability	3–10 reps
Inner Thigh Rotation *page 62*	small firm or stability	3–10 reps
Hamstring Curl *page 63*	large stability	1–10 reps
Isometric Hamstring Curl *page 64*	large stability	2–10 sec
Internal & External Shoulder Rotation *page 65*	small firm, or stability	3–15 reps
Wall Squat (avoid if you have heart issues) *page 66*	large stability	3–120 sec
Total-Core Stretch *page 67*	large stability	10–120 sec

stretch & relax

This routine is designed to be a "treat," to allow you to relax your mind and body. Try it after a warm bath accompanied by soft music. To gain the most from this routine, do as much or as little as you wish and, if you fall asleep, wonderful.

STRETCH & RELAX		
EXERCISE	**BALL**	**DURATION**
Spine/Neck Lengthener *page 68*	large stability	10–120 sec
Chest Stretch *page 69*	large stability	10–30 sec
Ab Stretch *page 70*	large stability and 2 small firm or hard	5–15 sec
Hip Flexor Stretch *page 71*	small firm or stability	1–30 sec
Inner Thigh Stretch *page 72*	small firm or stability	3–30 sec
Hamstring/Hip Release *page 73*	small firm or stability	3–30 sec

muscle release for active folks

This self-massage and muscle-release program is perfect after a hard day of playing, working in the garden or hunching over a computer. The moves in this routine can be selected based on whatever area is bothering you. There's no need to do every move—simply use this list as a menu. Do these moves for as long or as short as your body tells you. Some days your body will need more attention, other days less. Some days you have to avoid certain areas while other days nothing's off limits.

MUSCLE RELEASE FOR ACTIVE FOLKS		
EXERCISE	**BALL**	**TARGET**
Foot Massage *page 74*	small firm or hard	foot
Ankle Massage *page 75*	small firm or stability	foot
Knee Release *page 79*	small stability	knee
Calf Massage *page 80*	small firm or hard	leg
Inner Thigh Massage *page 78*	small firm or hard	leg
IT Band Massage *page 81*	small firm or hard	leg
Piriformis Release *page 82*	small firm or hard	leg
Hamstring Massage *page 76*	small firm or hard	leg
Quadriceps Massage *page 77*	small firm or hard	leg
Glute Massage *page 83*	small firm or hard	butt
Lower Back Release *page 85*	small stability	back
Upper Back & Shoulder Massage *page 84*	small firm or hard	back
Lat Release *page 86*	small firm or hard	back
Hand Massage *page 90*	small firm or hard	hand
Forearm Massage *page 91*	small firm or hard	arm
Biceps Massage *page 92*	small firm or hard	arm
Deltoid Massage *page 87*	small firm or hard	arm
Chest Massage *page 89*	small firm or hard	torso
Neck Release *page 88*	small firm or hard	neck
Combo Massage *page 93*	small firm	total body

PART 3

the exercises

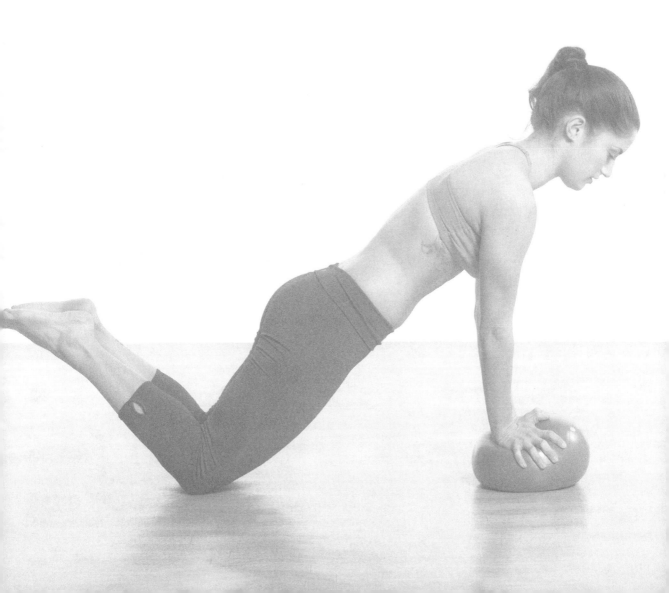

SUGGESTED BALL TYPE(S): small firm or stability

While this may appear to be a leg exercise, the emphasis is on engaging the abdominal muscles. The movements should be slow and purposeful.

1 Lie on your back with your knees bent and feet flat on the floor. Place a small ball between your knees and rest your arms alongside your body.

2 While maintaining a neutral spine, engaging your deep abdominal muscles and keeping the ball between your knees, slowly extend your right leg from the knee joint.

3 Slowly return to starting position and switch sides. Make sure you have proper neutral spine position each time.

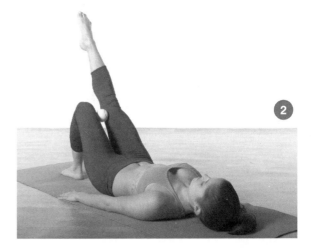

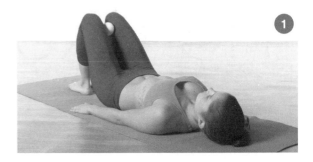

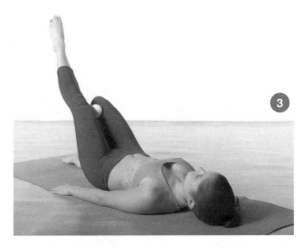

SUGGESTED BALL TYPE(S): small stability

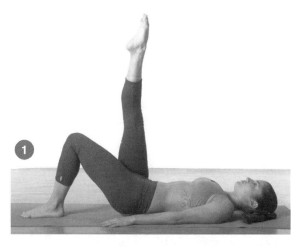

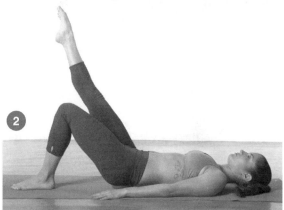

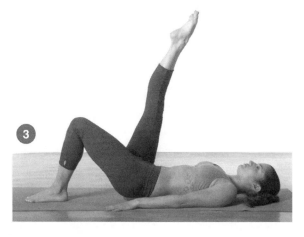

1 Lie on your back with your knees bent and feet flat on the floor. Place a small ball under your tailbone; adjust the ball so that you balance comfortably on it. Extend your arms along your sides for support. Once you've settled your weight into the ball, extend your right leg to the ceiling and point your toes.

2–3 Engaging your deep abdominal muscles to limit any hip movement, slowly and mindfully draw small circles on the ceiling.

Once you've performed the prescribed number of reps, switch sides.

SUGGESTED BALL TYPE(S): small firm or stability

This exercise is easier to perform if done on a smooth floor surface with stockinged feet.

1 Lie on your back with your knees bent and feet flat on the floor. Place a small ball under your tailbone; adjust it so that you balance comfortably on it.

2 While maintaining a neutral spine and engaging your deep abdominal muscles, slowly and mindfully slide your left heel forward along the floor. Avoid any side-to-side hip movement. Stop when you feel your lower back begin to arch.

3 Return to starting position and switch sides.

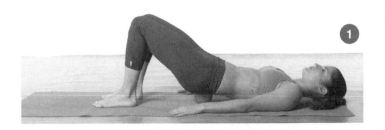

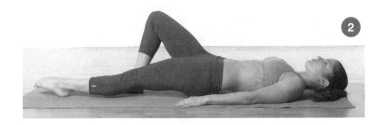

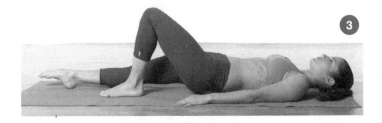

SUGGESTED BALL TYPE(S): small firm or stability

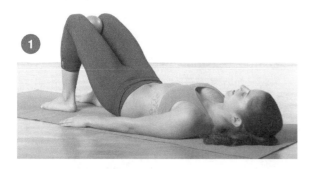

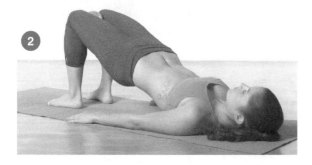

1 Lie on your back with your knees bent and feet flat on the floor. Place a small ball between your knees and rest your arms alongside your body.

2 Starting with your tailbone, slowly roll up your spine, feeling each vertebra contact the floor as you progress toward your shoulders. Stop when your hips are off the ground and you make a straight line from knees to neck.

Slowly roll back down to starting position, once again imprinting each vertebra into the ground.

arm swing

SUGGESTED BALL TYPE(S): small firm or stability

1 Lie on your back with your knees bent and feet flat on the floor. Place a small ball between your knees and extend both arms up to the ceiling with your palms facing each other. Your hands should be directly above your shoulders.

2 While maintaining a neutral spine, engaging your deep abdominal muscles and keeping the ball between your knees, slowly move one arm forward toward your hip and the other straight back alongside your head.

3 Slowly return to starting position and switch directions.

VARIATION: You may also move both arms in the same direction at the same time as well as open your arms out to your sides, but be especially mindful to maintain neutral spine.

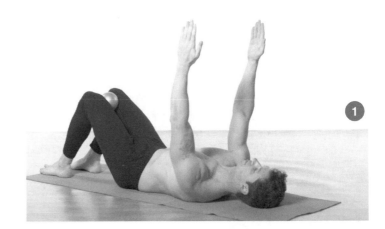

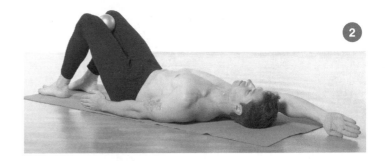

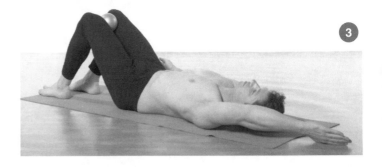

SUGGESTED BALL TYPE(S): small firm or stability

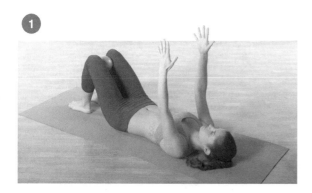

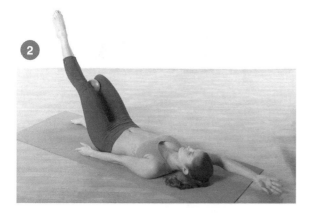

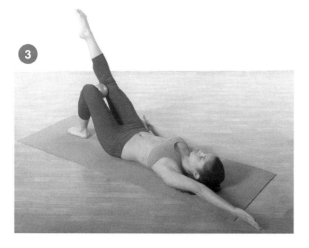

Pelvic control is critical in this exercise while speed nor quantity of reps are not important. Do not perform this exercise until you can perform the Leg Extension (page 22) and Arm Swing (page 26) correctly.

CAUTION: If you have an increase in lower back arch, you're not ready for this exercise.

1 Lie on your back with your knees bent and feet flat on the floor. Place a small ball between your knees and extend both arms up to the ceiling with your palms facing each other. Your hands should be directly above your shoulders.

2 While maintaining a neutral spine, engaging your deep abdominal muscles and keeping the ball between your knees, slowly move your right arm back toward your head and left arm toward your hip while simultaneously extending your left leg.

3 Return to starting position. Repeat with the opposite side.

SUGGESTED BALL TYPE(S): small firm or stability

These can also be considered half sit-ups. Focus on pressing your lower back into the floor, not on seeing how many reps you can do.

1 Lie on your back with your knees bent and feet flat on the floor. Place a small ball between your knees and place your hands behind your head in order to cradle and support your neck.

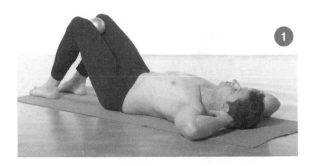

2 While contracting your abdominal muscles, inhale, tuck your chin to your chest and exhale while slowly lifting your shoulder blades off the floor. Hold for 1–3 seconds.

Inhale while slowly returning to starting position.

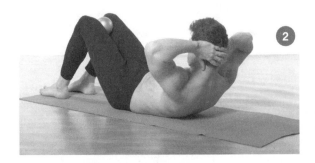

SUGGESTED BALL TYPE(S): large stability

This teaches you how to engage your core muscles and get used to performing movements on an unstable surface.

1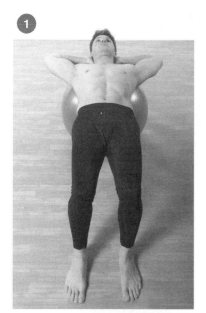

2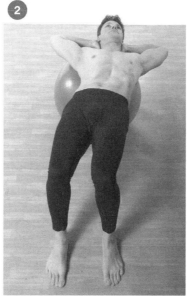

3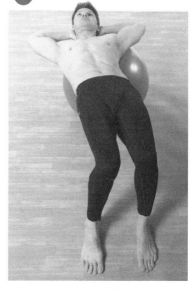

1 Sit on a stability ball and then slowly roll it toward your feet, moving your feet forward until the ball is comfortably beneath your upper back and head (you may also support your head with your hands). Your feet should be shoulder-width apart and knees bent 90 degrees.

2–3 Once you feel stable, gently roll left and right and recover your balance.

MODIFICATION: Hold your arms out to the sides for additional stability.

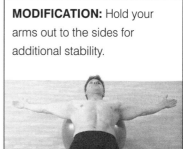

SUGGESTED BALL TYPE(S): large stability

1 Sit on a stability ball and then slowly roll it toward your feet, moving your feet forward until the ball is comfortably beneath your mid-back. Place your hands behind your head to support your neck. Your feet should be shoulder-width apart and bent 90 degrees.

2 Keeping your elbows wide and without pulling on your neck, slowly perform a half sit-up.

Slowly lower to starting position.

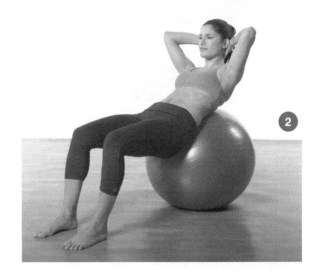

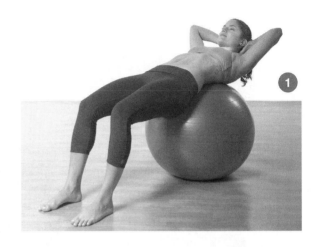

SUGGESTED BALL TYPE(S): large stability

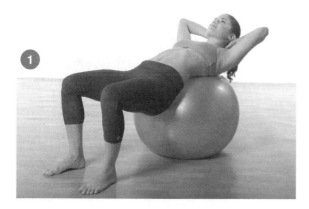

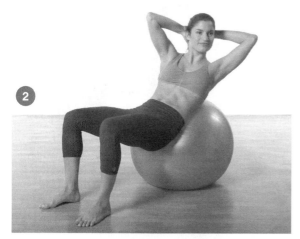

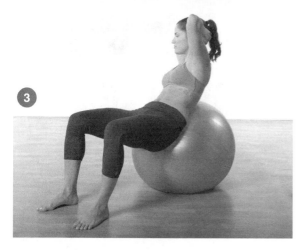

1 Sit on a stability ball and then slowly roll it toward your feet, moving your feet forward until the ball is comfortably beneath your mid-back. Place your hands behind your head to support your neck. Your feet should be shoulder-width apart and bent 90 degrees; always keep your knees aligned over your ankles.

2 Without pulling on your neck, curl up gently and attempt to bring your right elbow toward your left side.

3 Return to starting position and repeat to the other side.

SUGGESTED BALL TYPE(S): large stability

1 Sit on a stability ball and then slowly roll it toward your feet, moving your feet forward until the ball is comfortably beneath your upper back and head (you may also support your head with your hands). Your feet should be shoulder-width apart and knees bent 90 degrees.

2 Once stable, slowly lift your left foot 1–2 inches off the floor and hold for 15 seconds.

3 Return to starting position and lift the other foot.

Continue alternating.

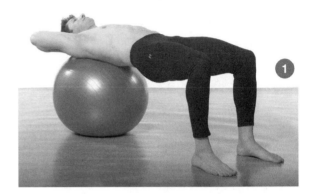

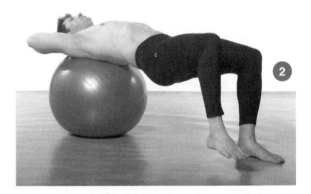

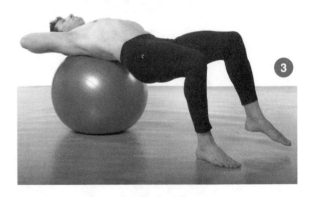

SUGGESTED BALL TYPE(S): large stability

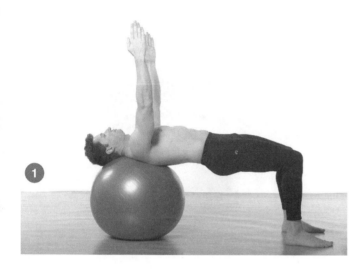

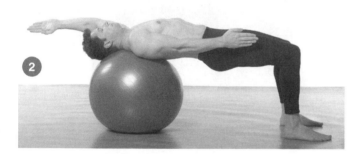

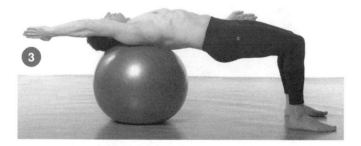

1 Sit on a stability ball and then slowly roll it toward your feet, moving your feet forward until the ball is comfortably beneath your upper back and head. Your feet should be shoulder-width apart and knees bent 90 degrees. Once stable, raise your arms up to the ceiling so that your hands are directly above your chest.

2 Engaging your core muscles, slowly move one arm down toward your hip and the other alongside your head.

3 Switch sides.

SUGGESTED BALL TYPE(S): large stability with small firm or stability

1 Sit on a stability ball and then slowly roll it toward your feet, moving your feet forward until the ball is comfortably beneath your upper back and head (you may also support your head with your hands). Your feet should be shoulder-width apart and knees bent 90 degrees; place a small ball between your knees.

2 Engaging your core muscles and keeping the small ball in place, slowly extend your right leg.

3 Carefully return to starting position and switch sides.

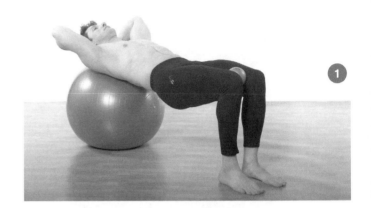

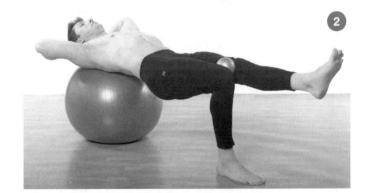

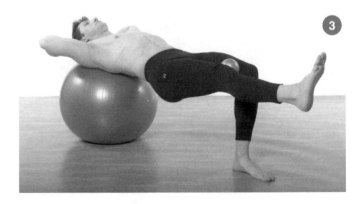

SUGGESTED BALL TYPE(S): large stability

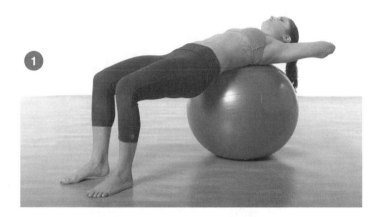

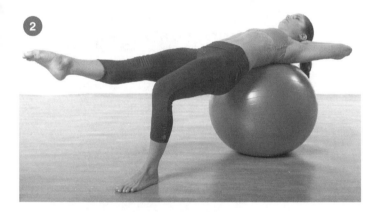

This is a challenging move.

1 Sit on a stability ball and then slowly roll it toward your feet, moving your feet forward until the ball is comfortably beneath your mid- to upper back. Place your hands behind your head to support your neck. Your feet should be shoulder-width apart and bent 90 degrees.

2 Once stable, lift and extend one leg until it's parallel to the floor.

Slowly lower to starting position and repeat with the other leg.

SUGGESTED BALL TYPE(S): small firm or stability

Focus on pressing your lower back into the floor, not on seeing how many reps you can do.

1 Lie on your back with your knees bent and feet flat on the floor. Place a small ball between your knees and place your hands behind your head in order to cradle and support your neck.

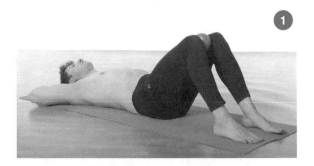

2 While contracting your abdominal muscles, inhale, tuck your chin to your chest and exhale while slowly lifting your shoulder blades off the floor and twisting your torso to bring your left elbow toward your right knee. Hold for 1–3 seconds.

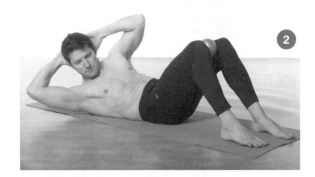

3 Inhale while slowly returning to starting position, and then repeat to the other side.

Continue alternating.

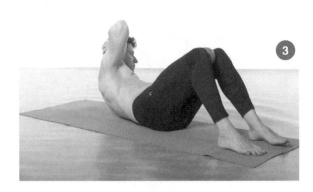

ADVANCED VARIATION: Bring your knees up until your legs form a 90-degree angle.

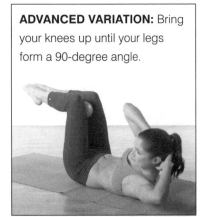

SUGGESTED BALL TYPE(S): large stability

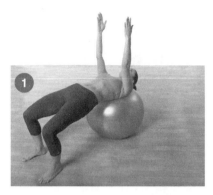

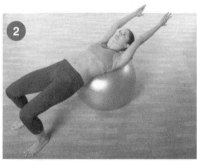

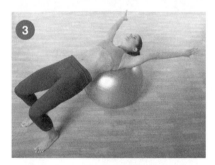

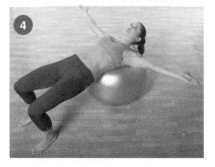

1 Sit on a stability ball and then slowly roll it toward your feet, moving your feet forward until the ball is comfortably supporting your upper back, neck and head. Your feet should be shoulder-width apart and bent 90 degrees. Extend your arms toward the ceiling with palms facing each other.

2 While engaging your core muscles, slowly and deliberately take both arms back by your ears, making your body look like an "I" from a bird's eye view.

3 Return to starting position and then slightly take your arms back and to the sides, as if making a "Y."

4 Return to starting position and then open your arms out to the sides to make a "T."

SUGGESTED BALL TYPE(S): large stability

1 Kneel in front of a stability ball and place your belly button on the ball so that the ball supports your midsection. Place your hands behind your head and extend your legs behind you, making a straight line from head to heels.

2 Keeping your head and neck neutral, squeeze your glutes and raise your chest off the ball. Don't come up too high.

Return to starting position.

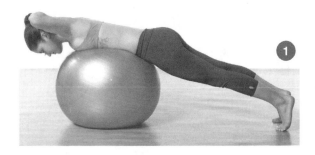

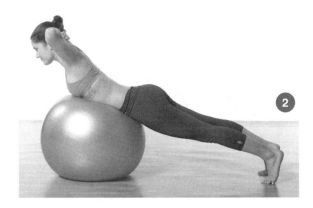

ADVANCED VARIATION: This can also be done from your knees.

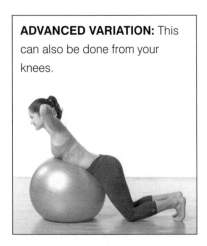

SUGGESTED BALL TYPE(S): large stability

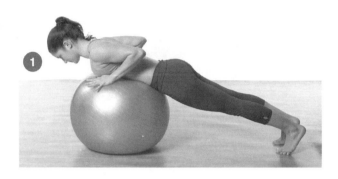

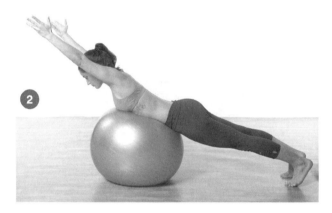

1 Lie facedown with your belly button on the middle of the ball and hands on the ball or on the ground in front of you. Extend your legs behind you with toes on the ground.

2 While maintaining neutral spine, slowly raise both arms and hold. Keep the motion smooth and avoid twisting your body.

Return to starting position.

MODIFICATION: This can also be done with one arm at a time.

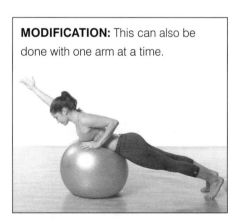

SUGGESTED BALL TYPE(S): large stability

1 Lie facedown with your belly button on the middle of the ball and hands on the ground in front of you. Extend your legs behind you with toes on the ground.

2 While maintaining neutral spine, slowly raise both legs and hold. Keep the motion smooth and avoid twisting your body.

Return to starting position.

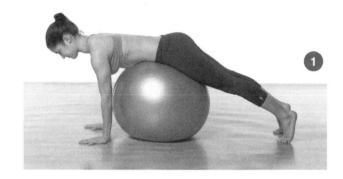

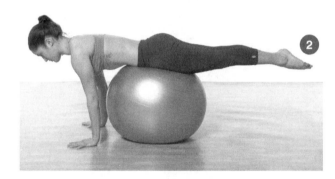

VARIATION: This can also be done with one leg at a time.

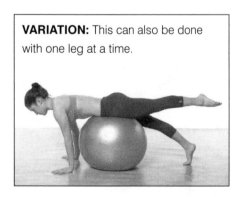

SUGGESTED BALL TYPE(S): large stability

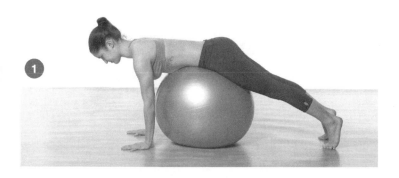

1

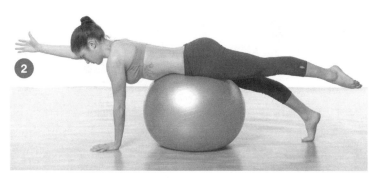

2

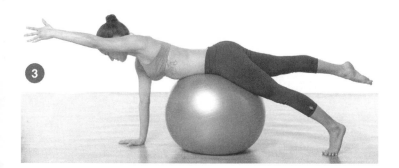

3

1 Lie facedown with your belly button on the middle of the ball and hands on the ground in front of you. Extend your legs behind you with toes on the ground.

2 While maintaining neutral spine, slowly raise your right arm and left leg. Keep the motion smooth and avoid twisting your body. Hold.

3 Return to starting position and repeat to the other side.

Continue alternating.

SUGGESTED BALL TYPE(S): large stability

This is a very challenging exercise. The area around you should be free of objects to avoid hitting them.

1 Lie facedown with your belly button on the middle of the ball and hands on the ground in front of you. Extend your legs behind you with toes on the ground.

2 While maintaining neutral spine, slowly raise both arms and legs and hold for up to 1 minute. Keep the motion smooth and avoid twisting your body.

Return to starting position.

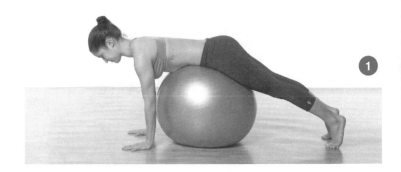

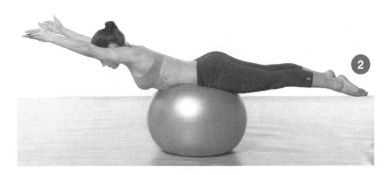

MODIFICATION: If you have shoulder issues, you may take your arms out to the sides in a "T."

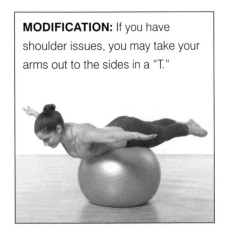

SUGGESTED BALL TYPE(S): medium or large stability

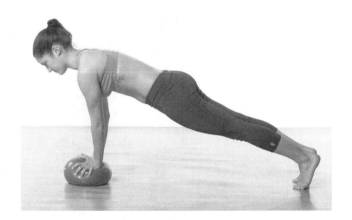

This exercise is about maintaining proper alignment. Make sure your ball is relatively firm.

THE POSITION: Place your hands on top of the ball and step your feet back until you're forming a straight line from head to heels. Engaging the gluteal muscles as well as the abdominal and upper torso muscles, hold for the prescribed amount of time. Lower to your knees to rest.

MODIFICATION: This can also be done with your knees on the floor.

VARIATION: Place your feet on the ball instead.

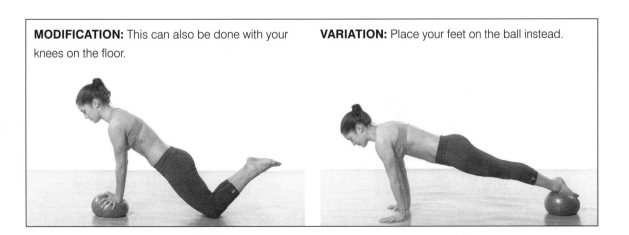

SUGGESTED BALL TYPE(S): medium or large stability

This exercise is about maintaining proper alignment, not how many push-ups you can do. Make sure your ball is relatively firm.

1 Place your hands on top of the ball and step your feet back until you're in a plank, forming a straight line from head to heels.

2 Engaging the gluteal muscles as well as the abdominal and upper torso muscles, lower your chest toward the ball.

Press yourself back up to starting position.

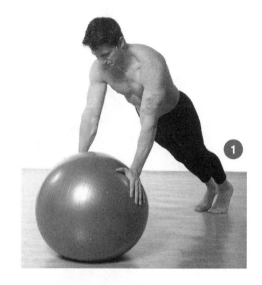

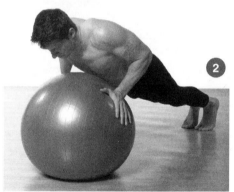

MODIFICATION: If this is too challenging, perform the push-up from your knees.

VARIATION: Place your feet on the ball instead.

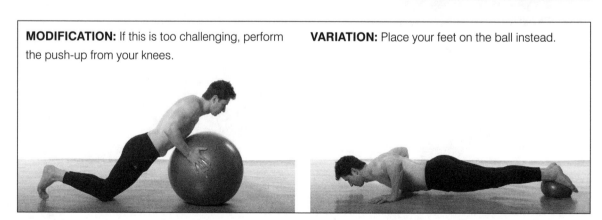

SUGGESTED BALL TYPE(S): medium stability or firm

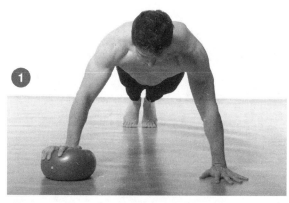

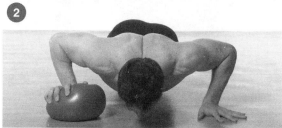

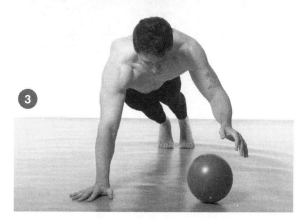

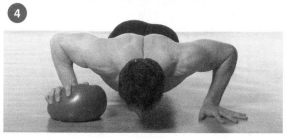

1 Place your right hand on top of a medium ball and step your feet back until you're in a plank, forming a straight line from head to heels.

2 Engaging the gluteal muscles as well as the abdominal and upper torso muscles, lower your chest toward the ground.

3 Press yourself back up to starting position and roll the ball to your left hand.

4 Perform a push-up with your right hand on the ball.

MODIFICATION: If this is too challenging, perform the entire exercise from your knees.

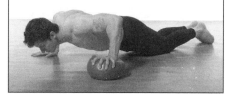

SUGGESTED BALL TYPE(S): large stability

Make sure your ball is relatively firm.

1 Place your hands on the floor and feet carefully on the ball, forming a straight line from head to heels.

2 Lift your rear end up into a pike position (inverted "V"). Hold for 15 seconds.

Return to starting position.

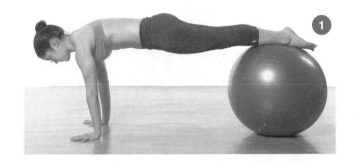

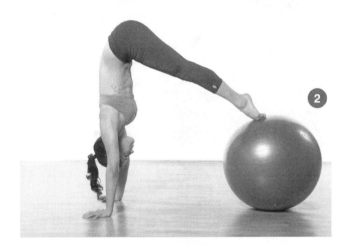

SUGGESTED BALL TYPE(S): large stability

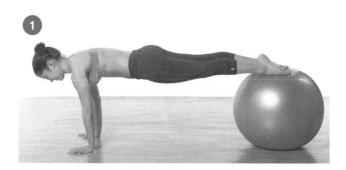

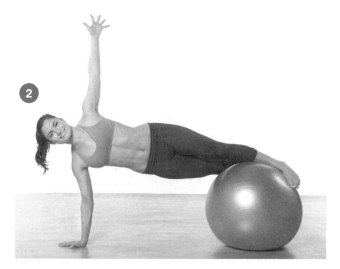

This is an extremely challenging exercise. Make sure your ball is relatively firm.

1 Place your hands on the floor and feet carefully on the ball, forming a straight line from head to heels.

2 Relying on your right arm to support you, slowly rotate your body to the left and extend your left arm to the ceiling.

Return to starting position and repeat to the other side.

SUGGESTED BALL TYPE(S): large stability

This is a very advanced exercise.
Proceed with caution.

1 Lie on your back with your arms
alongside your body and lower
legs resting on the ball.

2 Dig your heels into the ball,
gripping the ball between the
backs of your thighs and your heels,
and slowly pull your knees to your
chest, allowing your tailbone to
come off the floor.

Return to starting position.

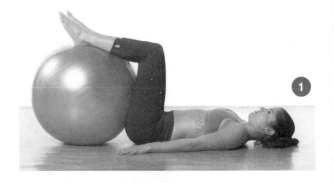

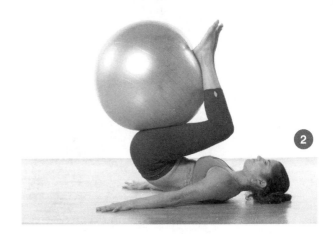

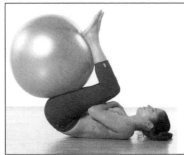

VARIATION: Place
your arms across
your chest and
perform the
movement.

SUGGESTED BALL TYPE(S): medium firm, hard or stability

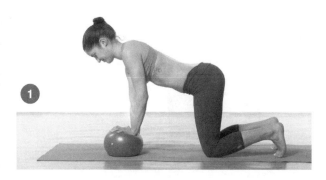

1

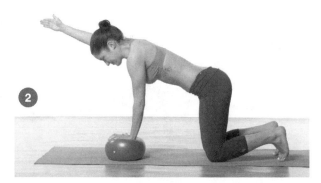

2

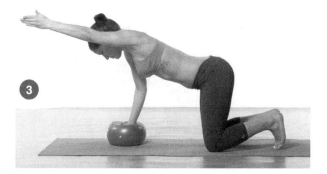

3

CAUTION: Avoid this move if you have wrist or elbow issues

1 Assume the hand and knee position (hands under your shoulders, knees under your hips, back neutral) and place a medium-sized ball under your left hand.

2 Engaging your core muscles, slowly raise your right arm until it's alongside your ear. Make sure not to twist your body. Hold.

3 Slowly return to starting position. Repeat, then switch sides.

SUGGESTED BALL TYPE(S): medium firm, hard or stability

CAUTION: Avoid this move if you have wrist or elbow issues

1 Assume the hand and knee position (hands under your shoulders, knees under your hips, back neutral) and place a medium-sized ball under your left hand.

2 Engaging your core muscles, slowly raise your right arm until it's alongside your ear and extend your left leg behind you; keep your hips level to the ground. Hold.

3 Slowly return to starting position and switch sides.

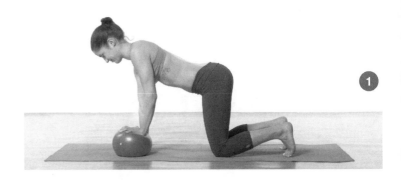

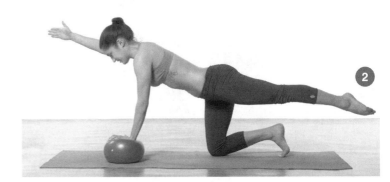

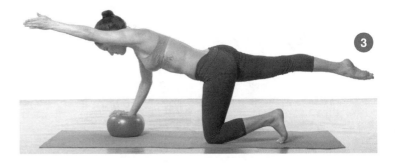

SUGGESTED BALL TYPE(S): large stability

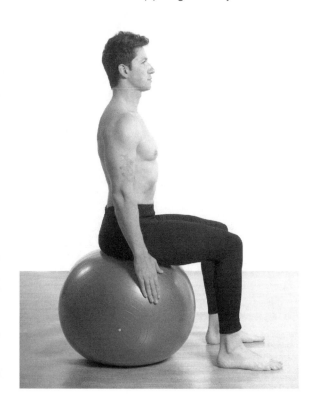

This move teaches you how to contract the abdominal wall and maintain neutral spine on an unstable surface.

THE POSITION: Sit on the ball and gently engage your abdominal muscles, locating neutral lumbar spine position. Focus on proper sitting alignment, with your head being lifted up by a string, chest up and out, and shoulder blades together.

SUGGESTED BALL TYPE(S): large stability

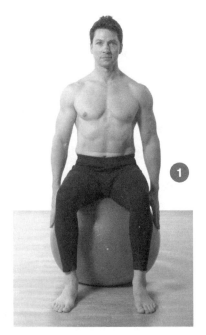

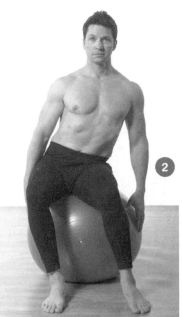

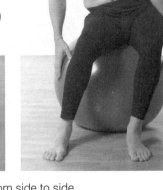

1 Sit on the ball and gently engage your abdominal muscles, locating neutral lumbar spine position and focusing on proper sitting alignment.

2–3 Gently roll your hips from side to side.

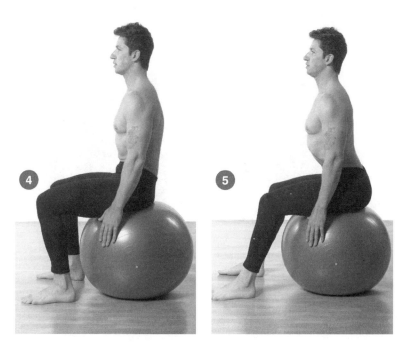

4–5 Now move the ball forward and backward by rolling your tailbone under you and then backward. Curving and arching of the lower back is tolerated in this situation.

Now move your hips in a clockwise direction. After a few clockwise rotations, move your hips counterclockwise.

SUGGESTED BALL TYPE(S): large stability

This exercise will progressively challenge your nervous system, teaching you how to contract the abdominal wall and maintain neutral spine on an unstable surface.

1 Sit on the ball and gently engage your abdominal muscles, locating neutral lumbar spine position. Focus on proper sitting alignment, with your head being lifted up by a string, chest up and out, and shoulder blades together.

2 Engaging your abdominal muscles to minimize movement, slowly lift your right foot off the floor approximately 3–5 inches and hold 3–5 seconds.

3 Slowly lower the foot and repeat with the other leg.

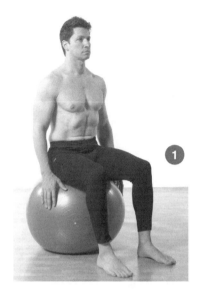
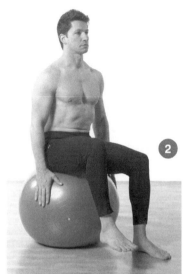
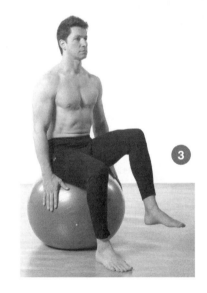

SUGGESTED BALL TYPE(S): large stability

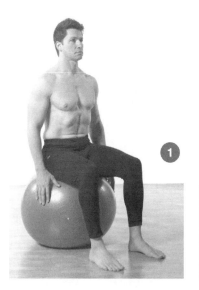

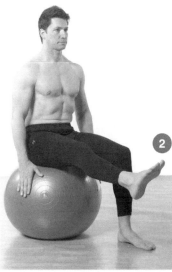

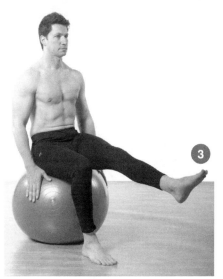

This exercise will progressively challenge your nervous system, teaching you how to contract the abdominal wall and maintain neutral spine on an unstable surface.

1 Sit on the ball and gently engage your abdominal muscles, locating neutral lumbar spine position. Focus on proper sitting alignment, with your head being lifted up by a string, chest up and out, and shoulder blades together.

2 Slowly lift your right foot off the floor and extend your leg from the knee joint. Hold 3–5 seconds.

3 Slowly lower the foot and repeat with the other leg.

ADVANCED VARIATION: Place a small ball between your knees.

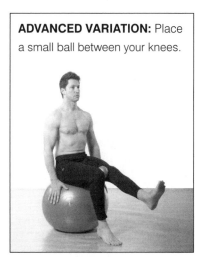

ball sit with leg extension & arm raise

target: abdominals

SUGGESTED BALL TYPE(S): large stability

This exercise will progressively challenge your nervous system, teaching you how to contract the abdominal wall and maintain neutral spine on an unstable surface.

1 Sit on the ball and gently engage your abdominal muscles, locating neutral lumbar spine position. Focus on proper sitting alignment, with your head being lifted up by a string, chest up and out, and shoulder blades together.

2 Slowly lift your right foot off the floor and extend your leg from the knee joint. Simultaneously raise your left arm up to the ceiling. Hold 3–5 seconds.

3 Slowly lower your arm and foot and repeat with the other side.

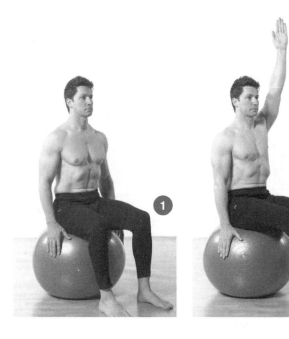

ADVANCED VARIATION: Place a small ball between your knees.

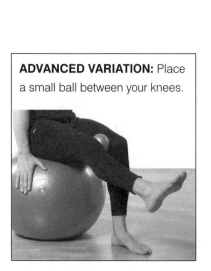

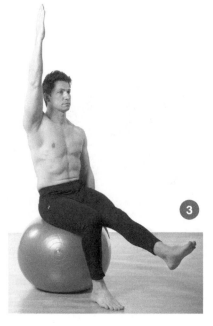

SUGGESTED BALL TYPE(S): medium firm, hard or stability

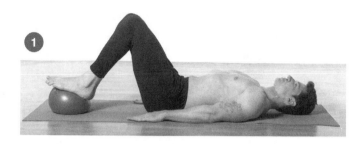

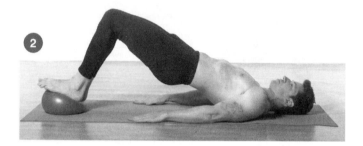

CAUTION: Be careful not to perform so many reps as to trigger a hamstring cramp.

1 Lie on your back with your knees bent and feet resting on a medium-sized ball. Place your arms alongside your body.

2 Press your feet into the ball to lift your pelvis off the floor; don't lift your butt so high as to arch your back. Hold 10–15 seconds.

Slowly lower to starting position and realign your spine before performing the next rep.

SUGGESTED BALL TYPE(S): medium firm, hard or stability

CAUTION: Be careful not to perform so many reps as to trigger a hamstring cramp.

1 Lie on your back with your knees bent and feet resting on a medium-sized ball. Place your arms alongside your body.

2 Press your feet into the ball to lift your pelvis off the floor; don't lift your butt so high as to arch your back. Hold 3–5 seconds while extending both arms to the ceiling, directly above your shoulders with palms facing each other.

3 Slowly move one arm forward toward your hip and the other back alongside your head.

4 Slowly return both arms to the ceiling and then switch directions.

Continue alternating.

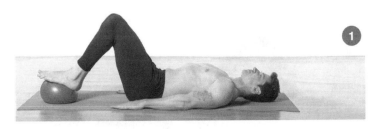

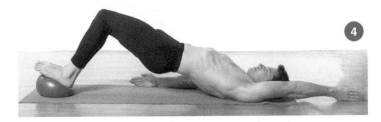

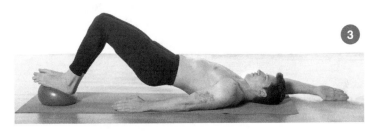

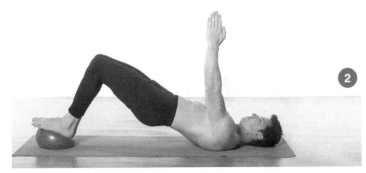

SUGGESTED BALL TYPE(S): medium firm, hard or stability

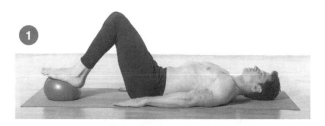

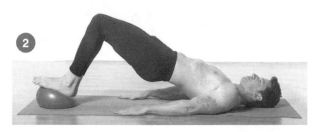

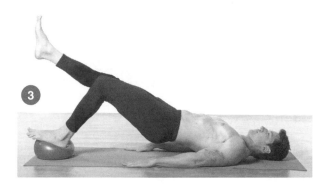

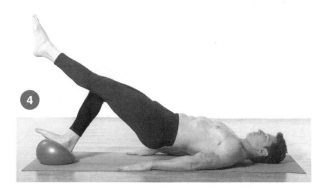

While this may appear to be a leg exercise, the emphasis is on engaging the muscles of the core. The movements should be slow and purposeful—avoid rapid leg motions.

CAUTION: Be careful not to perform so many reps as to trigger a hamstring cramp.

1 Lie on your back with your knees bent and feet resting on a medium-sized ball. Place your arms alongside your body.

2 Press your feet into the ball to lift your pelvis off the floor; don't lift your butt so high as to arch your back.

3 While engaging your abdominal muscles and maintaining neutral spine, slowly extend your right leg from the knee joint.

4 Slowly return your foot to the ball and repeat with the other leg.

VARIATION: For an additional challenge, place a small ball between your knees.

pelvic lift with arm lift & leg extension   *target: abdominals, butt, lower back*

SUGGESTED BALL TYPE(S): medium firm, hard or stability

This is a challenging exercise. Do not perform this until you can do Pelvic Lift with Arm Lift (page 58) and Stability Ball Pelvic Lift with Leg Extension (page 59) with perfect form.

CAUTION: Be careful not to perform so many reps as to trigger a hamstring cramp.

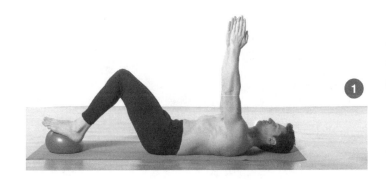

1 Lie on your back with your knees bent and feet resting on a medium-sized ball. Raise your arms up to the ceiling, directly above your shoulders with your palms facing each other.

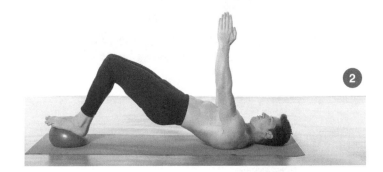

2 Press your feet into the ball to lift your pelvis off the floor; don't lift your butt so high as to arch your back.

3 While engaging your abdominal muscles and maintaining neutral spine, slowly extend your right leg from the knee joint while taking your left arm back alongside your head and your right arm forward toward your hip.

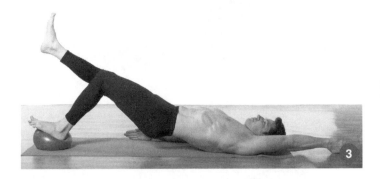

Slowly return to center and repeat to the other side.

> **VARIATION:** For an additional challenge, place a small ball between your knees.

inner thigh toner

SUGGESTED BALL TYPE(S): small firm or stability

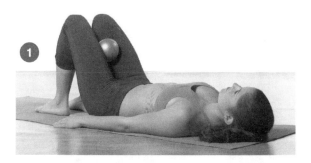

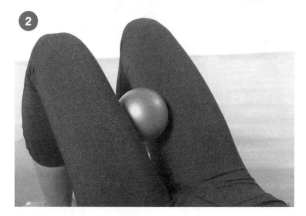

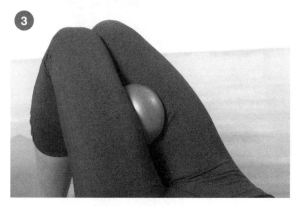

1 Lie on your back with your knees bent and feet flat on the floor. Place a ball between your thighs and rest your arms along your sides.

2–3 Engaging your abdominal muscles, quickly squeeze your legs together and then release, not allowing the ball to drop until you're done with your reps.

SUGGESTED BALL TYPE(S): small firm or stability

This movement requires 2 balls. It strengthens the inner thigh muscles and relieves hip tightness.

1 Lie on your back with your knees bent and feet flat on the floor. Place a medium-sized ball under your tailbone. Adjust the ball so that you balance comfortably on it. Once you've settled your weight into the ball, bring your knees to your chest and extend your legs to the ceiling. Place a second ball between your thighs.

2–3 Engaging your core muscles, slowly rotate your thighs around the ball, first inward and then outward.

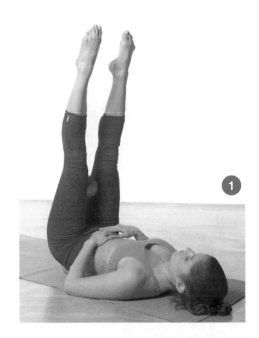

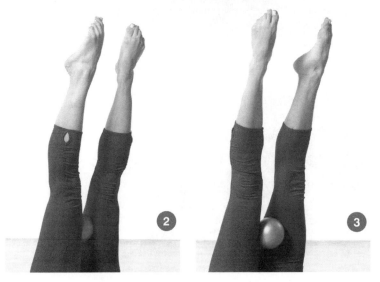

SUGGESTED BALL TYPE(S): large stability

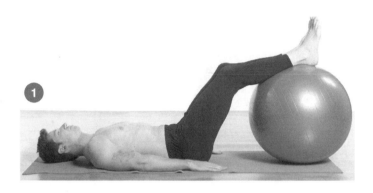

1 Lie on your back with your knees bent and feet resting on a large ball. Place your arms alongside your body.

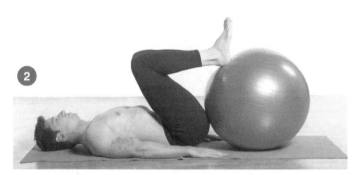

2 Press your heels into the ball while simultaneously rolling the ball toward your butt. Hold.

Extend your legs back to starting position. Make sure to return to neutral alignment before continuing.

ADVANCED VARIATION:
Perform the movement by lifting your hips off the floor and performing the curl without letting your butt return to the floor between reps.

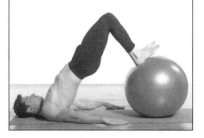

SUGGESTED BALL TYPE(S): large stability

This is an isometric exercise to tone the hamstrings.

1 Place your legs on top of the ball and rest your arms alongside your body.

2 Dig your heels into the ball and hold for 10 seconds, feeling the backs of your legs contract. Remember to breathe!

Slowly release.

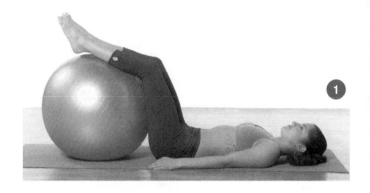

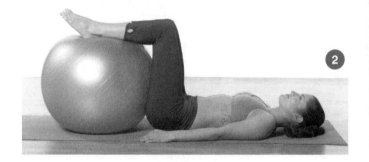

SUGGESTED BALL TYPE(S): small firm or stability

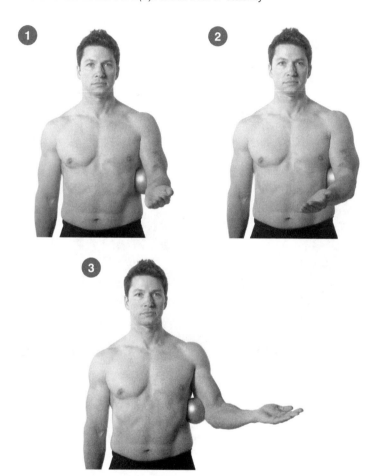

This can be done will standing or sitting.

CAUTION: Do not perform this exercise quickly as you may harm yourself.

1 Tuck a ball between your ribs and left upper arm, bend your elbow 90 degrees and turn your palm up. Stay mindful of engaging the deep muscles of the shoulder area.

2 Moving only your forearm, slowly bring your left hand toward your belly button.

3 Now slowly move your hand away from your body to the side. Do not force the movement past your comfort zone.

Repeat, then switch sides.

SUGGESTED BALL TYPE(S): large stability

1 Place a large ball between your upper back and a wall.

2 Bend your knees and lower yourself until your thighs are parallel to the floor (if possible). Hold.

Slowly return to starting position.

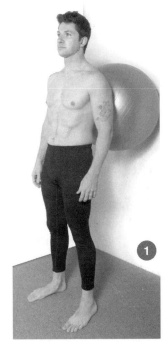

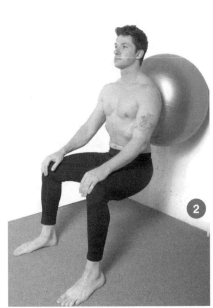

total-core stretch

SUGGESTED BALL TYPE(S): large stability

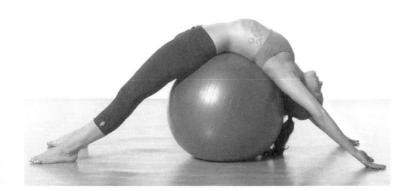

This is a very advanced stretch and requires a lot of back, chest and shoulder flexibility. Most people won't ever be as flexible as our model. If you decide to perform this move, proceed gently and slowly; avoid extremes.

CAUTION: Before doing this exercise, stand up and arch your back. If this feels uncomfortable, avoid this move.

THE POSITION: Sit on a stability ball and then slowly roll it toward your feet, moving your feet forward until the ball is comfortably beneath your mid-back. Your feet should be shoulder-width apart and bent 90 degrees. Start with a slight arch and move only within comfortable zones. If you feel comfortable, you may place your hands behind your head or extend your arms to the ground behind you; let your head be supported by the ball. Gently settle your weight into the ball, allowing your back to relax. Breathe slowly and fully.

GETTING OFF THE BALL: To get off the ball, support your head with your hands and slowly roll the ball toward your feet so that you may sit on the ground; move your feet forward accordingly.

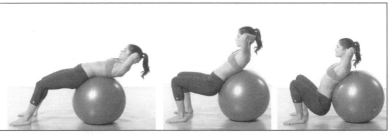

SUGGESTED BALL TYPE(S): large stability

This releases back tension and lengthens the spine and neck.

CAUTION: If you're pregnant or have stomach issues, speak to your health professional before doing this movement.

THE POSITION: Kneel in front of a stability ball. Drape your upper body over the ball, hugging the ball or placing your hands on the floor in front of you as necessary. Breathe slowly and fully.

To get off the ball, shift your weight back toward your hips so that you return to kneeling.

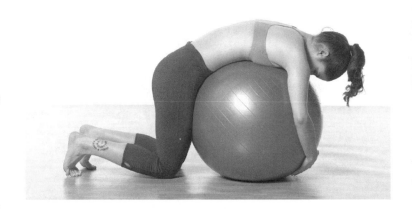

VARIATION: Straighten your legs to allow a wider range of release.

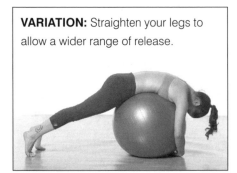

SUGGESTED BALL TYPE(S): large stability

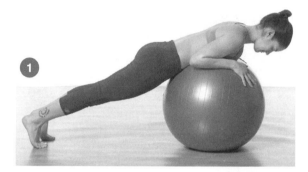

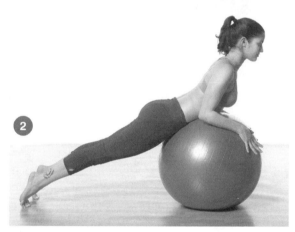

CAUTION: Be careful not to extend back too far; stay in your comfort zone.

1 Kneel in front of a stability ball and place your belly and chest on the ball. Rest your hands and forearms on the front of the ball. Extend your legs behind you, making a straight line from head to heels.

2 Keeping your head and neck neutral, gently raise your chest off the ball. Don't come up too high.

Return to starting position.

MODIFICATION: This can be done from your knees.

VARIATION: You may extend your arms back alongside your body to increase the stretch.

ab stretch

SUGGESTED BALL TYPE(S): large stability and 2 small firm or hard

This stretches the muscles of the abdominal area simultaneously along with upper torso.

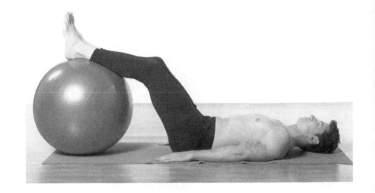

THE POSITION: Lie on your back and place your legs on top of a large ball. If you can tolerate it, place 2 small balls in a sock under your lower back. Place your hands anywhere they're comfortable (along your sides, under your head). Breathe and relax, allowing your abdominal area to elongate.

SUGGESTED BALL TYPE(S): small firm or stability

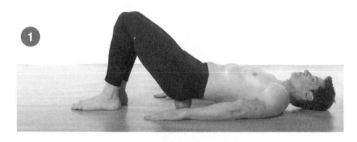

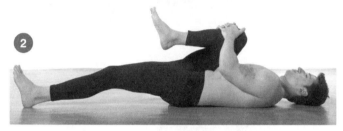

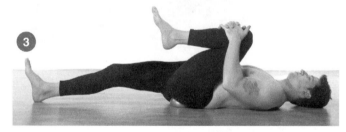

1 Lie on your back with your knees bent and feet flat on the floor. Place a medium-sized ball under your tailbone. Adjust the ball so that you balance comfortably on it.

2 Once you've settled your weight into the ball, inhale and bring your right knee to your chest and clasp your hands beneath your knee. Exhale and straighten your left leg as far as is comfortable. Hold, breathing slowly and fully, feeling the stretch in your extended leg.

3 Slowly switch sides.

72 **inner thigh stretch** *target: inner thighs*

SUGGESTED BALL TYPE(S): small firm or stability

1 Lie on your back with your knees bent and feet flat on the floor. Place a medium-sized ball under your tailbone. Adjust the ball so that you balance comfortably on it.

2 Once you've settled your weight into the ball, exhale and slowly let your knees drop open to the sides. Hold, breathing slowly and fully, feeling the stretch in your inner thighs.

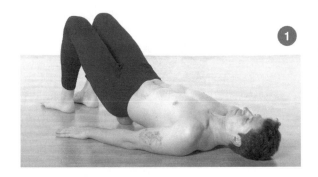

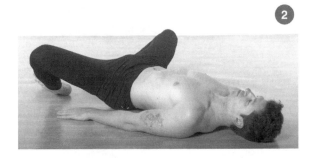

SUGGESTED BALL TYPE(S): small firm or stability

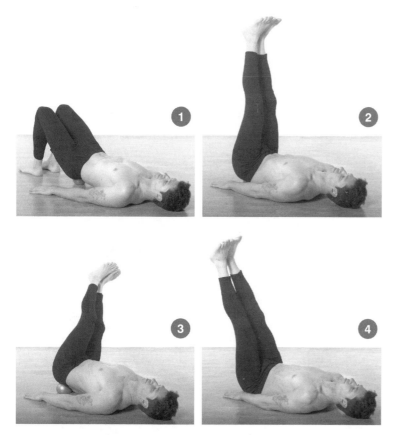

1 Lie on your back with your knees bent and feet flat on the floor. Place a medium-sized ball under your tailbone. Adjust the ball so that you balance comfortably on it.

2 Inhale and bring your knees to your chest and then exhale and extend your legs up to the ceiling, as if sliding your legs up an imaginary wall.

3 Keeping your legs together, gently shift your weight to your right hip. Hold, feeling the stretch in your hip.

4 Now gently shift your weight to your left hip and hold.

Repeat as necessary.

MODIFICATION: This can also be done against an actual wall.

SUGGESTED BALL TYPE(S): small firm or hard

This can be done while standing or sitting. If you have balance issues, standing by a wall or sitting is recommended.

1 Place a firm, small ball under the ball of your foot.

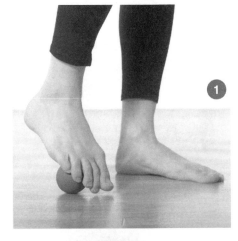

2 Roll the ball around under your entire foot and along the sides. Use your intuition to guide you on how hard to press and where/how long to roll. Breathe slowly and fully.

Switch sides.

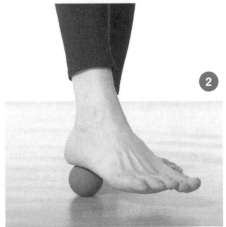

MODIFICATION: If rolling the ball underfoot is too painful, you can simply apply the right amount of pressure and hold, slowly moving the ball to another part of the foot once tightness has released.

SUGGESTED BALL TYPE(S): small firm or stability

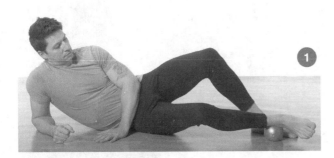

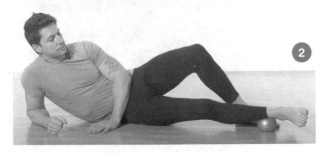

1 Sit on your left hip and position a ball under your anklebone.

2 Gently roll the ball under your ankle. Breathe slowly and fully.

Switch sides.

SUGGESTED BALL TYPE(S): small firm or hard

1 Sit upright in a chair and place 1 or 2 firm balls (in a sock) under the back of one leg.

2 Roll the ball(s) around under your thigh, from above your knee to under your buttock, controlling the pressure by shifting your weight. Use your intuition to guide you on how hard to press and where/how long to roll. Breathe slowly and fully.

Switch sides.

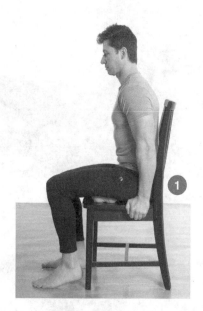

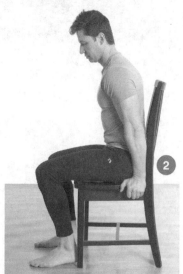

MODIFICATION: If rolling the ball is too painful, try slowly extending the leg, staying mindful of the pressure.

VARIATION: Sit on the floor with one or both legs extended. To make rolling easier, support yourself with your hands and/or bent leg to lift your butt off the floor.

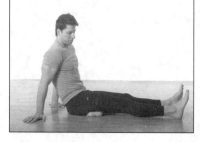

SUGGESTED BALL TYPE(S): small firm or hard

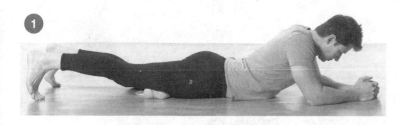

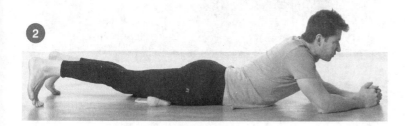

CAUTION: Avoid arching your lower back too much.

1 Lie facedown with your arms placed in a comfortable position to provide support. Place 2 small, firm balls (in a sock) under your thigh and just above your kneecap.

2 Roll the balls around under your thigh, controlling the pressure by shifting your weight. Use your intuition to guide you on how hard to press and where/how long to roll. Breathe slowly and fully.

Switch sides.

SUGGESTED BALL TYPE(S): small firm or hard

THE POSITION: Resting on your forearms, lie facedown with both legs extended. Bend your left leg and take your knee to the left side, opening up your hip. Place 1 or 2 firm balls (in a sock) under the inside of your left thigh. Gently roll the ball(s) around under your thigh, controlling the pressure by shifting your weight. Breathe slowly and fully.

Switch sides.

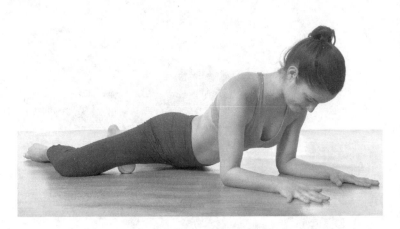

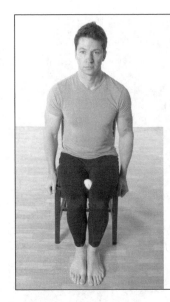

MODIFICATION: Sit comfortably in a chair and place a small ball between your thighs. Find a tender spot or trigger point and press your legs together to apply the ideal amount of pressure.

SUGGESTED BALL TYPE(S): small stability

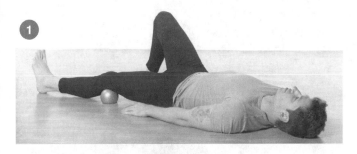

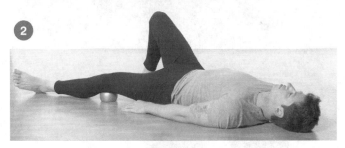

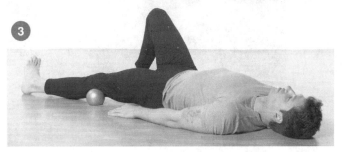

This can be done with both knees or one knee at a time. Make sure to use a soft, underinflated ball.

1 Lie on your back and place a small ball under one knee. Let your hip rotate if necessary.

2 Keeping your knee on the ball, let your knee roll outward. Relax and sink into the ball for 1 minute.

3 Now slowly rotate your knee inward. Relax and sink into the ball for 1 minute.

Remove the ball and let your leg rest on the floor before switching sides.

SUGGESTED BALL TYPE(S): small firm or hard

1 Sit on the floor with your legs extended and place your left ankle on top of your right. Place either 1 or 2 small balls (in a sock) under your calf muscles.

2 Apply gentle pressure into the ball, repositioning the ball(s) as needed. Breathe slowly and fully.

Switch sides.

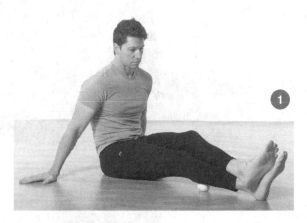

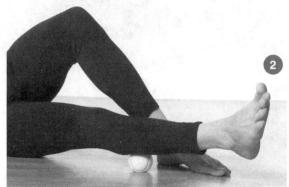

MODIFICATION: If crossing your ankles is too uncomfortable, uncross them.

SIDE CALF VARIATION: To cover the sides of your calves, you may need to roll onto your side, using your arms to adjust your weight as necessary.

VARIATION: To make rolling easier, support yourself with your hands and/or bent leg to lift your butt off the floor.

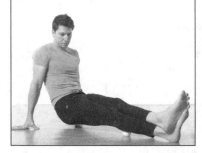

SUGGESTED BALL TYPE(S): small firm or hard

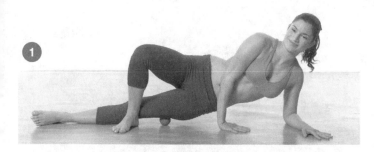

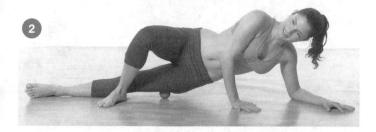

1 Sit on your left hip. Position either 1 or 2 small balls (in a sock) under your left thigh.

2 Supporting your weight as necessary with your hands/ forearms, roll the ball(s) along your outer thigh, from just above your knee to your hip. Breathe slowly and fully.

Switch sides.

SUGGESTED BALL TYPE(S): small firm or hard

1 Lie on your right side. Place 2 balls in a sock and position them under your right buttock.

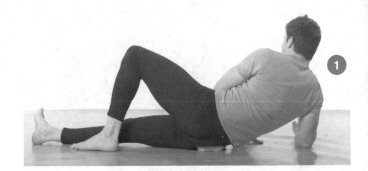

2 Using your arm to adjust your weight, apply the desired pressure. Breathe slowly and fully.

Switch sides.

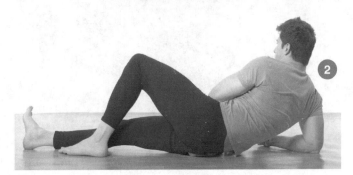

SUGGESTED BALL TYPE(S): small firm or hard

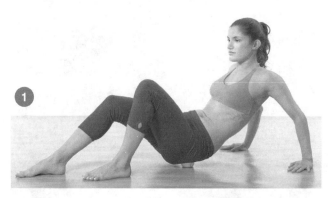

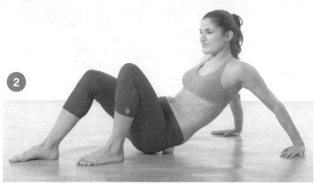

This can be done while sitting in a firm chair or on the floor.

1 While sitting, place a ball under one buttock. You may want to support yourself with your arms on the floor behind you.

2 Roll the ball around under your buttock, controlling the pressure by shifting your weight. Use your intuition to guide you on how hard to press and where/how long to roll. Breathe slowly and fully.

Switch sides.

VARIATION: To increase pressure, place one ankle on the opposite thigh.

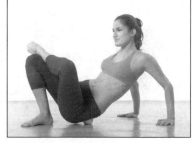

SUGGESTED BALL TYPE(S): small firm or hard

1 Stand with your back to a wall. Place either 1 or 2 small balls (in a sock) behind your back.

2 Gently move your torso around so that the ball(s) roll up and down your back along your shoulder blades and under your shoulders. Use your intuition to guide you on how hard to press and where/how long to roll; however, avoid rolling along your spine. Breathe slowly and fully.

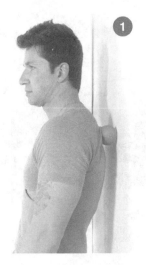
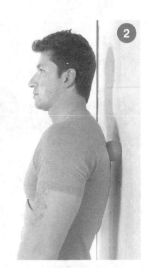

MODIFICATION: If rolling the balls is too awkward or painful, simply press your weight into the ball(s).

VARIATION: Perform this while sitting in a chair with a high, solid back or while lying on the floor with your knees bent and feet on the floor.

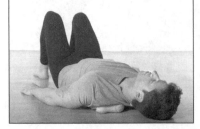

SUGGESTED BALL TYPE(S): small stability

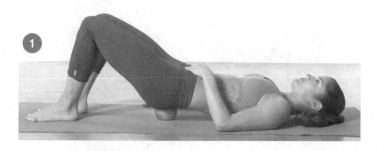

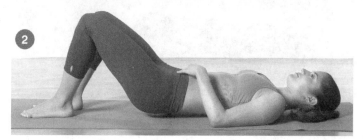

1 Lie on your back with your knees bent and feet flat on the floor. Place a medium-sized ball under your tailbone. Adjust the ball so that you balance comfortably on it.

2 Gently settle your weight into the ball, allowing your back to relax. Breathe slowly and fully.

VARIATION: You may also rock your hips from side to side, allowing your lower back to release more.

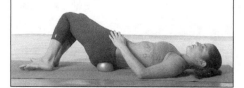

SUGGESTED BALL TYPE(S): small firm or hard

1 Lie on your right side with your head cradled by your right arm. Position 1 ball under your armpit.

2 Settle your weight onto the ball, adjusting the position of the ball with your other hand as necessary. Breathe slowly and fully.

Switch sides.

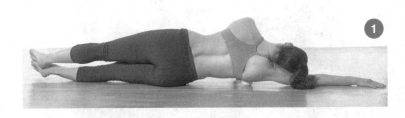

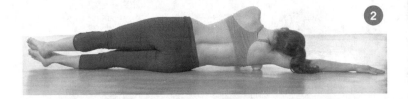

SUGGESTED BALL TYPE(S): small firm or hard

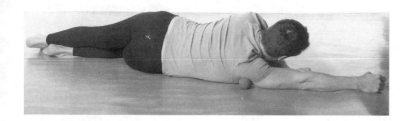

THE POSITION: Lie on your right side and position a small ball slightly to the rear of your shoulder. Settle your weight onto the ball and slowly roll the ball around your shoulder area. Use your right upper arm to adjust your weight as necessary. Breathe slowly and fully.

Switch sides.

SUGGESTED BALL TYPE(S): small firm or hard

This works best with 2 small balls in a sock.

THE POSITION: Stand with your back to a wall. Place the balls at the base of your neck. Gently press your neck into the balls and hold as desired. Breathe slowly and fully.

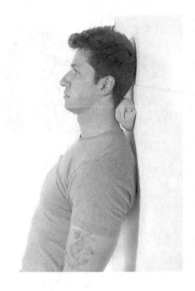

VARIATION: Perform this while sitting in a chair with a high, solid back or while lying on the floor with your knees bent and feet on the floor. If you're on your back, you may also gently turn your head left and right.

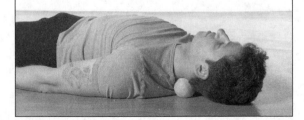

SUGGESTED BALL TYPE(S): small firm or hard

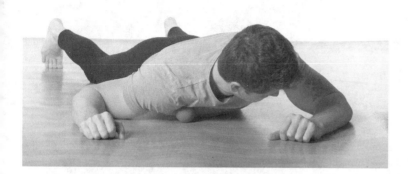

1 Position a ball at the intersection of your shoulder joint and chest and then lie facedown on the floor. Lift your body with your arms to control the pressure. Gently move your torso to roll the ball around that half of your chest. Use your intuition to guide you on how hard to press and where/how long to roll. Breathe slowly and fully.

Switch sides.

MODIFICATION: This can also be done while standing against a wall.

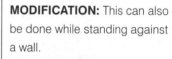
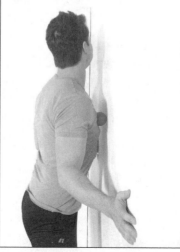

SUGGESTED BALL TYPE(S): small firm or hard

This can be done while standing, sitting or kneeling.

1 Place a small ball on a flat surface.

2 Roll the ball around under your hand, along the sides and on the back of your hand. Use your intuition to guide you on how hard to press and where/how long to roll. Breathe slowly and fully.

Switch sides.

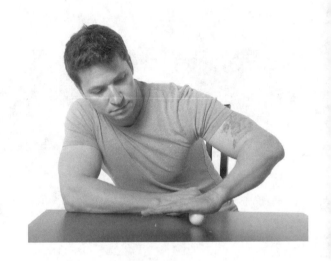

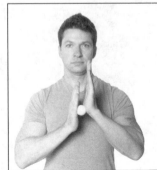

VARIATION: While sitting or standing, you can roll the ball between your hands, pressing your hands together to increase the pressure.

SUGGESTED BALL TYPE(S): small firm or hard

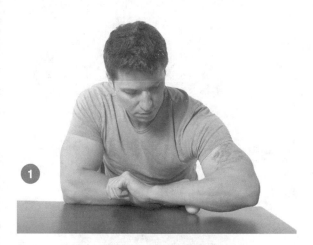

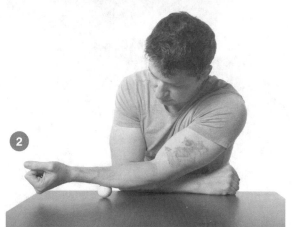

1 While seated, place a small ball on a flat surface.

2 Roll the ball around using your forearm—up and down as well as left and right. Use your intuition to guide you on how hard to press and where/how long to roll. Breathe slowly and fully.

Switch sides.

VARIATION: This can also be done while sitting or standing. Simply use your opposite hand to massage your forearm with the ball.

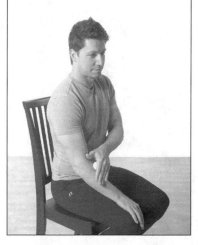

SUGGESTED BALL TYPE(S): small firm or hard

1 Lie facedown with your right arm extended to the side and left arm positioned in a comfortable location to offer support. Place a small ball under your biceps muscle.

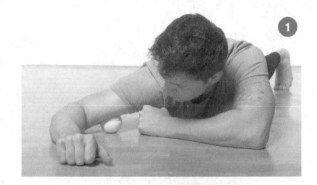

2 Roll the ball around under your biceps, controlling the pressure by shifting your weight. Use your intuition to guide you on how hard to press and where/how long to roll. Breathe slowly and fully.

Switch sides.

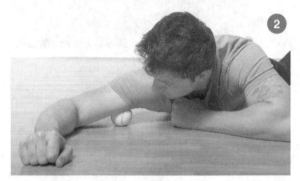

VARIATION: This can also be done while sitting or standing. Simply use your opposite hand to massage your biceps with the ball.

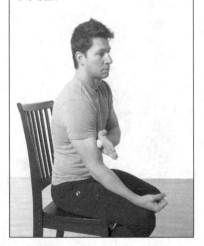

SUGGESTED BALL TYPE(S): small firm

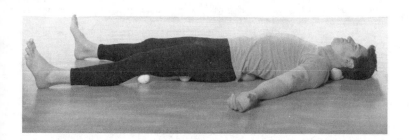

You'll need several balls to enjoy this one. Also, you may need a helper to place all the balls in the correct locations. Aim for 10 minutes of uninterrupted relaxation several times a week. Experts suggest that mindful relaxation is good for lowering blood pressure, reducing stress and encouraging creative thinking.

THE POSITION: Grab several balls. Dim the lights, turn on relaxing music and/or turn off all distractions then lie on your back. Place a ball under each calf muscle; place 2 balls (in a sock) under your hamstrings, 1 ball under your lower back area, 1 between your shoulder blades and 2 balls under your neck. If a thought comes to mind, acknowledge and release it with a breath.

VARIATION: To increase relaxation, you may tense a muscle for 5 seconds, inhaling slowly and exhaling even more slowly.

index

Acknowledgments

A giant appreciation goes out to Lily Chou, who has through the years been able to take my mumble jumble and turn it into simple and concise instructions. Lily, you're a wonderful partner! Special thanks also goes out to Claire Chun and Keith Riegert for their support and creative genius. Of course, this book could never have happened without the endless hours of work done behind the scenes by the production and marketing teams. Needless to say, my appreciation goes out to the staff at Rapt Productions and the skill and patience of models Michael Ciociola and Nadia Velasquez. Thank you to all at Ulysses Press for believing in me to write all the books we have done together—you're a great organization and I appreciate all you have done for me. Lastly, thanks to my wife Margaret for allowing me quiet time to work on this book—I owe you big time.

About the Author

Karl Knopf, has authored numerous books (including *Foam Roller Workbook*, *Healthy Hips Handbook*, *Healthy Shoulder Handbook*, *Stretching for 50+*, *Weights for 50+* and *Total Sports Conditioning for Athletes 50+*) that present safe and sane ways to improve the fitness of adults of all levels and ages. During his 40 years of teaching, he has served in many capacities with the fitness industry, from consultant on National Institutes of Health grants to advisor to the series Sit and Be Fit and to the State of California on disability issues. He has even worked with large health insurance companies to bring fitness programs to their members. Knopf has been featured in the Wall Street Journal and other national publications. He recently retired from Foothill College in Los Altos, California, where he taught adaptive fitness classes and directed the fitness therapy program. Knopf now serves as a director of fitness therapy and senior fitness programs for the International Sports Science Association.